MY BLOG TO BOOK
(2nd Edition)

Two Total Shoulder Replacements
- An (Im)patient's View
By Michelle Conway

https://shoulderreplacementblog.com

October 2015 to March 2017

Copyright Michelle Conway 2017

Michelle Conway asserts the moral right to be identified as the author of this work

All Rights Reserved

Faced with the prospect of a total shoulder replacement, I searched on the internet for someone to give me an insight as to what was to come. I drew a blank so I decided to write a blog to diarise the journey and hopefully to provide help to anyone else facing the same surgery in the future.

During the process, I learnt a lot of lessons, made some new friends and old friends supported me along the way with words of encouragement which I found to be extremely helpful. I decided to convert my blog into a book (now available from Amazon in paperback and kindle versions) which I myself found to be invaluable during my second total shoulder replacement, as I learned (the hard way), the right and wrong ways to do things the first time around!

Finally, I would like to thank Steve for all his love, help and support despite several visits by the "grumpy cow", everyone who has taken the time to read or comment on my blog, giving me words of support and encouragement during what seemed like a never ending journey and to my mam, who taught me as a very small child that "no matter how bad you feel there is always someone suffering more", and last but not least, thanks to the surgical team – because without them there would have been no story to tell.

Hope you enjoy reading.

If you want to read my blog, go to:
https://shoulderreplacementblog.com

CONTENTS

A Brief Introduction 1
The Beginning 5
The Procedure 7
The Gory Details 8
Hints and Tips for Surgery 10
A to Z of Hints and Tips 13
THE BLOG POSTS 17
    October 2015 17
    November 2015 17
    December 2015 30
    January 2016 50
    February 2016 57
    March 2016 64
    April 2016 68
    May 2016 71
    July 2016 73
    August 2016 75
    September 2016 77
    October 2016 79
    November 2016 93
    December 2016 101
    January 2017 108
    March 2017 109
Your Stories 112
The Gallery 119

October 2015
A Brief Introduction

I'm a 51-year-old female and next month I will undergo a total replacement of my left shoulder. Most people I've spoken to have never heard of such a thing and indeed I was surprised when I heard that this was possible. However, despite trawling the web for hours on end I have been unable to find anything which will tell me what I am letting myself in for. So hence this blog – to help not only anyone else who may have this procedure in the future, but also to remind myself of the journey I took, when it comes to having the other one done……

I am having the procedure under a nerve block alone – i.e. I will be awake for the op. Most people think that I must be mad but the doctor says that whilst I will feel pulling and tugging I will be pain-free. As it has been years since I was pain-free I want to be awake to experience that – if nothing else! I've been told I can take in my iPod so at least I can have the music to listen to instead of the grinding. I've had root canal surgery in the past so I'm sure I can cope. I'm not afraid of the surgery at all, however I am afraid of what comes afterwards. I'm a very independent person and I find it difficult to ask for help, something which I must do for a while after the surgery – especially the first two weeks when my arm is constantly in a sling. I'm going to turn into a right grumpy cow and I have already pre-warned those who will be affected!

I plan to update this blog once a week until the surgery and then frequently afterwards, so if anyone knows someone who has had this procedure already I would love to hear from them.

Comments

Tracy G (21-10 2015 at 11:55am)
*I will be closely following this blog and following your progress. We all need help in life at some time and seeing you do so much for everyone else it's only fair (karma ying and yang) that you have a couple of weeks following your Op being looked after. Hope the benefits of the Op far out way the negatives in the long run.
Best wishes from your best friend Tracy xxx*

Lorna March (21-10-2015 at 9:48pm)
I'm sure you will get through it fine, as you have done all your life no matter what has been thrown at you. You have always amazed me how strong you are even though you might not think it. I'm so proud of you keep your chin up sis. Love you x

Lilian Smith (23-10-2015 at 4:05pm)
*I completely agree with Lorna. You are so strong considering what you have been through. Keep strong my darling. Our love and prayers are with you all the time.
Aunt Lil.*

Lesley (23-10-2015 at 11:41pm)
*Good luck Michelle ... will be following your progress from over here in Oz!
Much love, Lesley x*

Marie (26-10-2015 at 2:36pm)
Best of luck Michelle, I will be following your updates and recuperation. xxx

Kathryn Main (14-04-2016 at 12:38pm)
Hi, I would like to give you my experience as someone with rheumatoid arthritis for 30 years and with multiple joint replacements. I had a full left shoulder replacement in the past 10 years and can reassure you that you will

cope. I did have it under a general anaesthetic but I have had other ops under epidural and would say that the recovery me is much quicker if you can avoid a general. Don't worry about the pushing and pulling you will get slightly sedated so you don't panic. Try to concentrate on your breathing to keep you calm. I appreciate you are an independent person but remember people do like to help and if it makes your life slightly easier then let them. As for the sling the time will go quickly. I remember taking it off and resting the arm on a pillow for a change. Afterwards you will have to do physio. I had to set up a pulley on the side of the door surround to help with lifting of the arm. Hopefully if you do your physio then you will gain a good amount of mobility in your arm and you will be pain free. That is the goal. I think you have the right mind-set to achieve it. Good luck and I'm sure it will go well. If you want to discuss it further let me know and I will be happy to help.
Kind Regards, Kath

Peta (20-04-2016 at 7:20pm)
I had right shoulder replaced a couple of years ago and left will be done this June. Right shoulder now pain-free with excellent movement. I did some physio exercises pre-op and was very diligent post-op with exercises. Swimming gently within four weeks and do recommend getting good physio and advice. Can't wait until left shoulder is done and a good night's sleep! Start practising early doing tasks with 'wrong' arm. I am left-handed so this me will find things a little more awkward but I will cope! Good luck.

ME (20-04-2016 at 7:28pm)
I had left replacement in November unfortunately I tore the rotor cuff tendon four weeks later and was in surgery on Christmas Eve for a repair. It's taken a long me to get back to where I was before the tear but I'm hoping to get the right arm done later this year. Good luck with yours please let me know how you get on.

The Beginning

For some years, I have been experiencing shoulder pain. It started in my right shoulder many years ago when I was on the rowing machine in the gym and I 'pulled it'. To cut a long story short the pain came and went, I had physio and saw a chiropractor – both of which helped for a while. About two years ago the pain started in my left shoulder, however unlike the pain in the other one which came and went, this was almost constant. Day to day tasks became increasingly difficult and I had to stop knitting squares for charity – something which I miss immensely.

Many visits to the GP resulted in many changes in medication in an attempt to manage my pain. Endless sleepless nights resulted in depression, extreme tiredness and yet more visits to the GP, who eventually referred me to the shoulder clinic where x-rays showed severe osteoarthritis in both shoulders. At this point I discovered that physio and injections were not going to help my problem and that the only real solution would be surgery. I was given an appointment to see the consultant and in the meantime, I did some searching on the web (as you do) and discovered that there was in fact a number of things they could do.

One of these was a procedure called arthroscopic sub acromial decompression. This procedure removes the inflamed bursa and some bone from the irritated area around the rotator cuff tendons. By removing this issue, more space is created for the tendons and the inflammation often subsides. Somehow I thought this would be the answer to my problem but was shocked when the consultant said that this procedure would not fix my problem and the best thing to do was a total joint replacement. I was shocked to say the least, whilst I knew this was always a possibility I somehow thought they may be able to try something less drastic and invasive first!

So, after a Q and A session with the consultant I decided to go ahead with the surgery.

The Procedure

Shoulder Replacement Surgery
(see http://orthopedics.about.com) updated 08 September 2014)

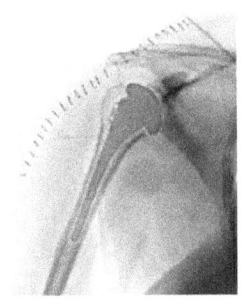

"Total shoulder replacement surgery alleviates pain by replacing the damaged bone and cartilage with a metal and plastic implant. The shoulder joint is a ball and socket joint, much like the hip joint. The ball is the top of the arm bone (the humerus), and the socket is within the shoulder blade (scapula). This joint allows people an enormous range of motion at the shoulder. When shoulder replacement surgery is performed, the ball is removed from the top of the humerus and replaced with a metal implant. This is shaped like a half-moon and attached to a stem inserted down the centre of the arm bone. The socket portion of the joint is shaved clean and replaced with a plastic socket that is cemented into the shoulder blade.

Shoulder replacement surgery lasts about two hours. The incision for the surgery is along the front of the shoulder joint and usually about four to six inches long. The surgery is most commonly done under general anaesthesia".

So, I hear you ask, why the hell do you want to stay awake? Well like I said in the introduction, it's been so long since I've been without pain I want to be awake to experience it! In addition, it means a quicker recovery time and with all the other medical conditions I have going on, it's probably the safest route to take - or maybe it's just morbid curiosity.☺

The Gory Details

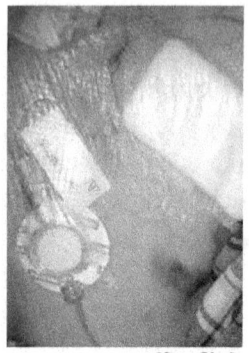
Nerve Block

I was away from my bed for five hours but that included travelling time and time spent in recovery afterwards.

First I had obs done and a cannula fitted. Then I had the nerve block injection in my shoulder which was a bit painful and uncomfortable. I still have a tube in my shoulder which is slowly administering some drugs from a small ball device which I will be carrying around in a little bag for two and a half days. It's all taped to my shoulder and up my neck so that and the sling means I'm not very comfortable.

I was given extra steroids because I have Addison's disease, then wheeled into theatre where there was a bit of shuffling onto another bed before the surgeon did final checks and put on what looked like a space helmet or bee keeper type thing. They then rigged high screen and taped it tightly around my shoulder. I was given a mild sedative, put my iPod on and off we went.

I can honestly say I felt no pain but it sounded like some serious carpentry was going on behind the screen. I heard a drill and what sounded like a saw and felt a bit of vibration when the hammer came out but felt no connection to my body at all; it was almost as though they were hammering on a table next to me. Throughout the operation the anaesthetist and nurses kept a close eye on me, checking that I was comfortable and doing obs.

Someone on the other side of the screen was holding my hand up the whole time and when they finished my arm was put in a sling across my body but weirdly I could still feel my hand I the air and felt no connection to my arm at all.

I then went into the recovery room where I was given a lovely warming inflatable blanket to raise my temperature before taking more obs and returning me to the ward in time for visiting.

The anaesthetist said she was really pleased at how well it went as not many patients manage a total joint replacement without a general anaesthetic. She said my positive attitude helped and I couldn't help but feel quite pleased with myself. ☺

Hints and Tips for Surgery

For anyone who is due to have similar surgery I recommend a bit of forward planning.

Pre op

- Practice going up and down the stairs using only one arm – the handrail will be on the wrong side at some point.
- If taking regular medication, put enough into containers for two or three weeks to avoid having to push pills out of foil packets.
- Practice all tasks normally done with other hand at least four weeks before operation e.g. wiping 'important little places', putting on lipstick, brushing teeth/hair and drinking cups of coffee.
- Practice eating using cutlery in the 'opposite hand', if you are having surgery on the dominate arm then you may need to use the other one for a while.
- Try to do some simple exercises until date of operation.
- Practice getting up and down from a chair and bed not using operated arm.
- Have a dental check–up to ensure no loose fillings or crowns.
- Get eyelash and eyebrow tint or consider getting hair cut short – if you can bear it.
- Get a manicure and pedicure week before op – but no nail polish.

Clothing

Firstly, think about what you wear each day, ladies will need to think about purchasing some front fastening bras as it will be some time before you can fasten your own around your back. This is fine as long as you are not larger than a D cup – which is where I found my first problem. After spending hours trailing around shops and browsing on–line, I managed to get myself a couple from Asda Direct. In addition, consider the following items:

- Jogging bottoms, or elasticated waisted trousers (or a size bigger than usual) are another 'must have' – it's so much easier going to the loo with one hand if you don't have to fiddle with buttons and belts – or wear skirts.
- Slip on shoes or boots with zips are much easier than laces.
- Shirts which button up the front are great for the first couple of weeks when you may find it difficult to get dressed.
- Night–wear needs to be considered as you will be wearing the sling in bed at night so I advise that you wear a nightshirt (or pyjamas) with a collar to stop it rubbing your neck, again button–up will be easier for the first week or so.
- Cloak for a coat if winter.
- Loop ear–rings (studs won't work).

Safety Issues

- Look at bathroom carefully. Would a temporary grab handle help get in and out of shower/bath? Do you need an additional non–slip mat in shower?
- Bedding – duvets can be heavy. Would you be better with a sheet plus a light fleece blanket?
- Soft pillow vertically on operated side to rest shoulder/elbow in sling and ensure you don't turn onto the shoulder during sleep.
- Leaving hospital and travelling in car: use a small hand towel under seat belt if it has to go over the operated shoulder – or sit in the back of the car on the opposite side.

- Shower cape – wound dressings are waterproof but additional protection might be considered. These are re–useable and keep shoulder dry under shower. Or hairdressing waterproof cape.

Post–op

- Post op Exercises: do in front of mirror to ensure that you keep your shoulder down.
- Ice, Ice, Baby – before and a lot after your shoulder replacement operation.
- Use small flannel for 'wall push' exercises to protect hand/arm/wrist.
- Tea towels make good bibs post operation when eating!
- Purchase E45 (cheaper) or Bio oil to use on scar four days AFTER removal of stitches.
- At one of my physio sessions one of the exercises involved the use of a shoulder pulley – which you can make yourself but I found one on www.amazon.co.uk which has had great reviews and cost under £8. I found this easy to use once I found a door which I could leave closed whilst I used it.

In addition, think about what you can do to make life easier once you come home from hospital, anything you can cook and freeze in advance will be useful and don't forget you can buy pre–prepared vegetables from the supermarket. I was actually very surprised at the quality and variety of those available and will probably use some of them again in the future.

A to Z of Hints and Tips

A AMAZON – sells ice-band, shoulder pulleys and other useful items.

B BATHROOM – look at bathroom carefully. Would a temporary grab handle help get in and out of shower/bath? Do you need an additional non–slip mat in shower?

BEDDING – duvets can be heavy. Would you be better with a sheet plus a light fleece blanket?

C CLOTHING – easy to put on and take off. Cloak for a coat if winter.

D DENTIST – have a dental check up to ensure no loose fillings or crowns.

E E45 – purchase E45 (cheaper) or Bio oil to use on scar four days AFTER removal of stitches.

EARRINGS – loop ear–rings (studs won't work).

EATING – learn to use cutlery with your 'other' hand.

EXERCISE – follow instructions from physio, don't over–do it!

EYELASH and eyebrow tint – before surgery.

F FRONT–FASTENING BRA – no explanation needed!

G GETTING UP – practice getting out of a chair and out of bed.

H HAIR – consider getting hair cut short – if you can bear it, or use a hairband.

I ICE – Ice, Ice, Baby – before and a lot after op.

ICE BAND – can be purchased from several online retailers.

J JOGGING BOTTOMS – elasticated waist or size bigger.

K KITCHEN – use pre–prepared vegetables from supermarket.

L LEARN – to do tasks with the opposite hand, especially if surgery is on dominant shoulder.

M MEDICATION – if you are taking regular medication, put enough into containers for two or three weeks to avoid having to push pills out of foil packets.

MOISTURISE – skin on shoulder to ensure that skin is not too dry, and lower legs which will get very dry whilst wearing the surgical stockings

N NIGHTWEAR – needs to be considered as you will be wearing the sling in bed at night so I advise that you wear a nightshirt (or pyjamas) with a collar to stop it rubbing your neck, button–up will be easier for the first week or so.

O OUTDOORS – wear sling for the first few weeks, take care travelling on buses.

P PILLOWS – a soft pillow vertically on operated side to rest shoulder/elbow in sling and ensure you don't turn onto the shoulder during sleep.

PRACTICE – all tasks normally done with other hand at least four weeks before operation e.g. wiping 'important little places', putting on lipstick, brushing teeth and drinking cups of coffee.

Q QUESTIONS – don't be afraid to ask questions, physio, consultant or any other medical staff.

R ROTOR CUFF – this is <u>very fragile</u>, beware of sudden sharp movements.

S SHIRTS – which button up the front, are great for the first couple of weeks when you may find it difficult to get dressed.

SHOES – slip on shoes or boots with zips are much easier than laces.

SHOULDER PULLEY – used for exercise post op and can be purchased from Amazon.

SHOWER – consider a shower cape, wound dressings are waterproof but additional protection might be considered.

SKIRTS – may be easier to wear instead of trousers (toilet visits).

STAIRS – practice going up and down the stairs using only one arm – handrail will be on the wrong side at some point.

T TRAVELLING – in car: use a small hand towel under seat belt if it has to go over the operated shoulder – or sit in the back of the car on the opposite side.

U UNDERWEAR - almost impossible to wear without help, go bare if you dare!

USELESS and UPSET – is how you may feel, its expected and its temporary.

V VANITY – no chance, you will look and feel like a ragamuffin for at least a couple of weeks.

W WELL DONE – congratulate yourself on achieving every small milestone, you will feel better.

WIPES – face wipes, deodorant wipes and toilet wipes – very handy.

X X–RAYS – if you are curious, ask to see your before and after x–ray's when you attend your post op out–patients' appointment.

Y YOU – will be tired, frustrated and grumpy – live with it, it won't be for long.

Z ZZZ – some people find it easier to sleep in a reclining chair in the early days' post op. If sleeping in bed as normal, more pillows may be required, especially under the operated shoulder.

THE BLOG POSTS

October 2015

Three weeks to go.... (27-10-2015 at 8.10am)
I'm not feeling great today, I've had a rotten cold virus for well over a week now and the cough is keeping me awake at night. Unfortunately, this gives me too much time to think, to think about horror stories of what can go wrong and to remind myself that I wouldn't be doing it at all if I could carry on living with the pain. Six years ago I was in the same predicament while I awaited surgery on my spine and I know from my own experience that things are going to get a LOT worse before they get better. But get better they will – as long as I do the exercises and don't try to hang out the washing!

November 2015

Two weeks to go.... (03-11-2015 at 8.05am)
Now that it's getting closer, the time seems to be dragging and I just want it done and finished. Unfortunately, my cough is showing no signs of shifting any time soon and it could delay the surgery if it is still hanging around in two weeks.

In preparation, I've been practicing going down the stairs backwards as I will need a handrail and it is on the 'wrong' side going down – sideways doesn't seem to work as easily. I'm also keeping a bag upstairs so that I can carry things downstairs if I need to. Lots of things are going to be difficult without the use of both arms. Silly things you take for granted like putting in contact lenses, earrings, doing your own hair and making a cup of tea – and don't even get me started on wiping my bum!

Comments

Lesley (03-11-2015 at 8:41am)
Mmm ... putting in contact lenses... That would be hard as you need one hand to keep your eye open and the other to put it in. Hope you've got a pair of glasses! As for wiping your bum, I can send you over a cork from last weekend's champagne bottle if you like?

One week to go.... (10-11-2015 at 7.49am)

The surgery date is on the horizon but for some reason I feel it will be postponed. Unless my health is up to standard then it won't go ahead. My cough has almost gone following a course of antibiotics but my foot injury is still causing some concern, although it's been almost two months since my accident. A physio appointment today and another check at diabetic clinic on Monday will hopefully rule out any possible problems in this area.

Comments

Lesley (10-11-2015 at 8:10am)
Got my fingers crossed for you Michelle. It would be awful psyching yourself up for it and then having to postpone. x

Two days to go.... (15-11-2015 at 12.19pm)

I've spent the weekend catching up and wondering when I will be able to do normal day-to-day tasks again. Some things will be impossible, but who knows maybe I'll master the art of putting my socks on with one hand - even sending a text will be a challenge with one arm in a sling. However, tomorrow I need to go back to the diabetic clinic so they can check on my foot injury - which bizarrely has been OK up until this morning and now it is feeling a bit strange. I'm going to try not to think about it too much but if they think that there is anything to worry about then the surgery may be delayed. This is the last thing I want - after building myself up for the last six weeks it would be awful to be postponed at the last-minute.

Comments

Lesley (15-11-2015 at 7:53pm)
Been thinking about you Michelle, wondering if things are still on track. Hope all goes to plan. Good Luck! Oh yeah, just thought, how are you going to update us on your blog with one hand? You will need a secretary!

ME (15-11-2015 at 8:20pm)
Thanks Lesley but where there's a will, there's a way. Maybe I can get Steve to temp for me until I get used to it.

Claire B (16-11-2015 at 9:01pm)
Hi Michelle! I'll be thinking of you tomorrow - can Steve do an update on your blog to let us know how it went? Try to think of the big picture - it will be worth it in the end. This is the first blog I've ever read - thanks for leading me into the 21st century!

ME (16-11-2015 at 9:07pm)
Thanks Claire, I've never read or written a blog either so it's a learning experience and great therapy when you know people actually care. I'm hoping to be able to do updates myself, although they may be short and take me ages, it's not like I'll be doing much else!

Today's the day.... (17-11-2015 at 6.48am)
So, the 'big day' finally arrives. I'm feeling ok at the moment, but I'm sure that will change once we get into the car to leave. I've done as much as I can to prepare myself for this day, I just hope it's enough, if not then I just have to muddle along and do the best I can. I would like to thank those of you who posted comments or sent me texts of support, these are really helpful and I'm sure it will help in my recovery if I know people are waiting for the next blog

update. Special thanks to Steve who is my rock, I'd have never got as far without him, and I'm sorry if I turn into a grumpy cow today.

I'm not afraid of the surgery, even staying awake isn't bothering me, however I am afraid of the recovery. The long journey to hell is about to begin so wish me luck and I hope to blog soon...

Comments

Lesley (17-1-2015 at 7:00am)
Good luck - thinking of you and looking forward to your next update! xx

Deanna Van der Velde (17-11-2015 at 8:09am)
All the very best to you be thinking about you

What utter chaos! (17-11-2015 at 9.59am)
Arrived to be greeted by the fire alarms going off and none of the fire wardens could tell us anything other than we had to wait. When they finally let us through the usual way to the ward was blocked off and we had to take a diversion around what seemed like the entire hospital, before we got to the ward. Maybe it's an omen and I should make my escape now before they put the ID tag on…..

On my way home.... (17-11-2015 at 11.36am)
No op today - major trauma means all today's procedures are cancelled. Told that waiting list manager would be in touch to rearrange. Don't know when so I guess I just have to wait - again. I did have a feeling last week and the chaos this morning just enhanced that feeling. I feel at a bit of a loose end now, nothing to do at home except have a coffee and put my contact lenses in. ☹.

Comments

Lesley (17-11-2015 at 8:35pm)
OMG! So your intuition was right, one way or another. So sorry for you, getting all psyched up... what a bloody let down.

New date.... (17-11-2015 at 1.02pm)
Just as I was sitting here thinking that I'd pretty much cancelled my life for the rest of the year, the phone rang and now the op is back on for Friday this week. I've not unpacked yet so I guess this morning was a bit of a rehearsal. I'll probably be in hospital over the weekend though but I can live with that. So more next week...

Comments

Deanna Van der Velde (17-11-2015 at 1:13pm)
Just enjoy the next couple of days xx

Lesley (17-11-2015 at 8:36pm)
Oh that's great news, not long to wait then. Staying 'tuned ....

Today's the day - again! (20-11-2015 at 6.24am)
Well here we go again, I need to check into the ward by 7.30am so just a few things to do before I leave - I only wish that having a strong coffee and a bacon sarnie was one of them! I've had to fast since midnight and I've had the WORST night this week - not helped by the fact that Steve was involved in a road traffic accident on his way home from work last night. Fortunately, he is OK, which is more than can be said for the car which they say is probably a write off. I slept really badly, with a new thing to worry about now as well as being unable to get comfortable lying in any position.

So part of me is wondering whether or not to postpone so that I can be here in case anything happens to Steve while

I'm away and the other part wants to carry on and see if it happens today. I just hope that if it is going to happen today I'm one of the first on the list.

Watch this space ....

Comments

Lorna March (20-11-2015 at 7:53am)
Morning flower I couldn't sleep last night either for thinking about you both. You know there is no way Steve would let you postpone this. Good luck, see you tomorrow xxx

One step closer.... (20-11-2015 at 7,59am)
Looks like it's happening this afternoon. The surgeon has just drawn a lovely picture on my arm ☺

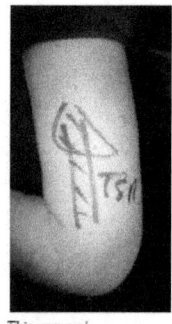

This way up!

Comments

Lorna March (20-11-2015 at 8:05am)
Oh well better late than never I suppose. I thought you would have been down first this morning x

ME (20-11-2015 at 8:07am)
Me too, I've told them I'm diabetic so they'll be keeping a close eye on me.

Operation over, ready for next challenge....
(20-11-2015 at 7:49pm)
Surgery done under nerve block only as planned and went really well. Anaesthetist said I can have a gold star. Will update you all more tomorrow. Thanks for your support ☺

Comments

Lorna March (20-11-2015 at 9:25pm)
Well done Michelle so proud of you x

Lesley (20-11-2015 at 10:51pm)
Hurray! One down one to go then!
Sending all good wishes from Oz and hope Steve's feeling ok x

A new chapter.... (21-11-2015 at 7.04am)
I will add a new page later with all the gory details and just make small posts during the day. Nerve block is wearing off and pain is AWFUL, as I have the same problem in my right shoulder I didn't appreciate just how much work it would have to do and how exhausting and frustrating every small task would be. There have been tears overnight and I'm sure there will be more later.

Comments
Deanna Van der Velde (21-11-2015 at 7:58am)
Today will be a bit of a blur. Try and rest / sleep as much as you can.
Will say a little prayer for you in Shul xx

Tracy G (21-11-2015 at 10:05am)
Aww you poor thing .... Don't be afraid to ask for more Meds for the pain Shelly and stay strong sweetheart .... You're the first person I know who's had a shoulder replacement and so I can't give you any advice but the only thing I'd say is don't sit in pain make sure you let them know you need more meds or stronger ones at least. Take care darling thinking of you xxx

Lesley (21-11-2015 at 10:12am)
Aww ... hang in there. Your poor thing... my Dad had both hips replaced (twice) and always wore the 'good' one out whilst recuperating from surgery on the 'bad' one, so I hear what you're saying. Sending good vibes your way x

Lorna March (21-11-2015 at 12:01pm)
Ah no bless you, yeah make sure you keep topped up with pain relief don't suffer in silence ASK!!! See you soon for a big hug xx

Making a little progress.... (21-11-2015 at 4.34pm)
Today I've managed to go to the loo myself, brush my teeth and eat my lunch totally unassisted. Such small steps but at least they are steps in the right direction.

The physio has been and we went through how to remove the sling and which exercises I need to do. I have to do them three times a day but wear the sling after getting dressed and after exercises. I think the hardest part will be trying to relax my shoulder as the taped in nerve block tube means that I'm trying to minimise the tape pulling on my neck by holding my shoulder up. Should be much easier when it's removed - probably on Monday.

Comments
Deanna Van der Velde (21-11-2015 at 6:40pm)
So much for resting. This is day 1 towards the future.

Lesley (22-11-2015 at 4:53am)
Yay go you! Guess it's a bit like when you have a baby ... amazing what you can do with one hand ☺

Bruised and aching.... (22-11-2015 at 6.24am)
Slept much better last night but you wouldn't believe how much I ache today. More nerve block is probably wearing off and I guess the right arm aches as it's having to do almost everything including occasionally lifting what feels the huge weight of my left arm. My back aches too - I could do with a nice soak in the bath but that's not going to happen any time soon. Got some very impressive bruising appearing on my arm - photos later.

Comments

Lesley (22-11-2015 at 6:42am)
Must say you're getting very good at this one-handed typing!

Tracy G (22-11-2015 at 9:28am)
First few days are always the worst Hun but as I knew ...you would always adapt to every situation your faced with and I just hope the pain and the aches subside soon so you have some decent sleep etc. xxx thinking of you

Another step forward.... (23-11-2015 at 1.47am)

Yesterday was awful - when I woke up my hand was completely numb and it pretty much stayed that way all day. Various medics came to look at it and the decision was made to temporarily switch off the nerve block as sometimes when they stop the pain this can happen. It was planned to switch it back on after a couple of hours but the day went on with no feeling at all.

Needless to say, there were tears and lots of self-pity but after five hours there was a twitch and it was slow improvements from then. It's now the middle of the night and I'm thrilled to report that I may have turned a corner. I'm so excited I've just been down to nurses' station to tell them the good news and squeeze both hands with almost equal force. Now I just need to make sure I don't overdo things as anyone who knows me will know what I'm like.☺

Comments

Lesley (23-11-2015 at 1:54am)
*Aww .. big hugs from Oz coming your way!
Glad your hand has gone back to normal, that would have been real scary x*

On my way home - again.... (23-11-2015 at 4.31pm)

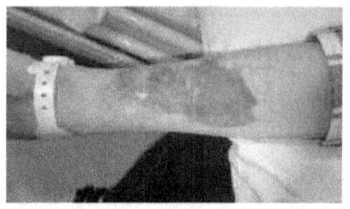

The cannula and nerve block have been removed, x-ray and blood tests have been done, and I've got a lovely bruise on my 'good' arm.

Now I'm just waiting for discharge papers and return appointment then I can go home - then the really hard work starts. Steve's on his way and I've managed NOT to pack my bag although all my stuff is out of the locker and lying on the bed. I've also dressed myself (slowly) apart from my shoes which are in the holdall which I'm unable to open with one hand. I will do a tidy of my blog tomorrow with another update. Thanks to everyone who has taken the time to read it, with special thanks to those who have followed with words of encouragement over the last week and all the lovely medical staff who have looked after me over the last three days. ☺

Comments

Deanna Van der Velde (23-11-2015 at 4:43pm)
Well done now you can do things at your own pace.
Each day is a day away from the op xx

Tracy G (24-11-2015 at 9:42pm)
Glad your home Hun .... and I'm sure you will find new ways to adapt around the house. Hope you get a better rest at home ... Thinking of you xxx big hugs

My first day home.... (24-11-2015 at 1.13pm)
I'm pleased to be home but it's so frustrating having to ask for so much help when I'm usually very independent. I'm really struggling to manage with just the right arm, especially as this is also painful and stiff due to the osteoarthritis in that shoulder. On a plus side I'm getting

really good at coming down the stairs backwards something I need to do as the handrail is on the wrong side for coming down. Unfortunately, I'm finding the general effort of just managing with one hand really tiring so I'm off for a nap, I will ask Steve to take a picture of my bruised left arm later so check this blog again tomorrow for a peep.

My neck is red and itchy where the nerve block was taped to it - but hopefully that will settle soon.

After today I will only post if there is something to report otherwise this blog will get very boring. Please sign up for email updates if you want to follow my progress. Thank you all x

Comments

Claire B (26-11-2015 at 10:08pm)
Michelle, you are AMAZING! I can't believe what you have been through, with local anaesthetic, and with your other health issues.
It's also amazing what doctors can do these days. I know the coming days and weeks will be very frustrating and uncomfortable, but try and remind yourself just how far you've come and what you've achieved.

Day 5 post op.... (25-11-2015 at 3.45pm)

As promised yesterday here is a picture of my bruised left arm - which is a LOT better believe me! There is more bruising around the elbow than the shoulder but apparently this is normal.

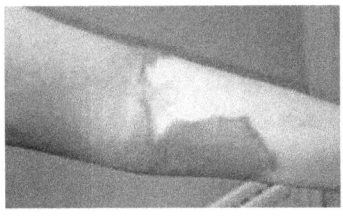

I said I would only post if there was something to report – and today is definitely one of those days. I have managed to put in my contact lenses today and you would not believe

how much better I feel just having them in. I am also feeling less nauseous today as I'm slowly reducing the codeine and am pleased to report that I feel more aching and stiffness in my shoulder than actual pain - but I'm prepared for the fact that this may not be the case tomorrow.

So fingers crossed it's all going in the right direction ☺

Comments

Deanna Van der Velde (25-11-2015 at 5:34pm)
Glad things are going in the right direction Remember a day at a time.

Lesley (25-11-2015 at 8:04pm)
Great news! One question ... why is the bruising on your arm? Is there some on your shoulder too?

ME (26-11-2015 at 2:07pm)
Very little bruising on shoulder, I think it's travelled down my arm as it was held up at right angle to my body during the whole surgery.

Adrienne Ross (26-11-2015 at 7:58pm)
Glad you are making progress. I go for my pre-op tomorrow, but I haven't got a definite date yet. We are coping, but we miss you! x

One step back.... (27-11-2015 at 2.32pm)
The Grumpy Cow has arrived! I'm not at all happy today, my wound is itchy and it pricks (sign of healing), I have a lot of pain under my arm and around my back which I am blaming in wearing the sling 99% of my life and my legs itch from the awful surgical stocking which I've to wear for ANOTHER FIVE WEEKS!!!! In addition, I've no energy and basically can't be bothered with anything - so you are lucky to get this update.

Still it's only been a week I suppose ☹

Comments

Deanna Van der Velde (27-11-2015 at 3:24pm)
Stick the telly on and watch something daft. It's cold and miserable outside and just started to rain so stay warm x

Claire B (27-11-2015 at 7:50pm)
Hi! There's going to be ups and downs - and a lot of frustration! I suspect that day to day improvements are not going to be that noticeable, but I bet that in a week you'll be amazed how much you've improved. Your body has been through a big trauma; I'm not surprised you're tired. Just hang in there (easy for me to say!). x

Tracy G (27-11-2015 at 10:06pm)
Chin up sweetheart it's early days and things can only improve in me .... It's ok to be a grumpy cow after everything you are going through and just remember everyone's routing for you xxx big hugs

Lesley (27-11-2015 at 10:20pm)
Hey there Grumpy! Guess it's only natural for 'two steps forward, one step back' to happen. Take the opportunity to revel in laziness and not feel guilty. I would! xx

Steve (28-11-2015 at 5:47am)
*Sometimes you might be a grumpy cow but you're my grumpy cow and I love you.
I hope I'm helping as best I can xx*

Claire B (28-11-2015 at 9:45pm)
I love your comment Steve. It made me go aaahhhh ☺

A nice bath.... (29-11-2015 at 6.16pm)
For some reason I decided that it would be a good idea to try and have a bath today. I managed to get in facing the wrong way then do a half turn before lowering myself into

the bath - I had to do it this way so that I could support myself with the 'good' arm. So, I had my bath, feeling quite pleased with myself until I came to get out .... oh dear!

I realised that my 'good' arm wasn't strong enough to pull myself up. So we emptied the bath and I tried to turn over onto my knees. Unfortunately, I kept slipping and by this time I was starting to worry. Then I had a brainwave and asked Steve to fetch a rubber mat which we got under me so I could turn over onto my knees before standing up. Just as well I had room to do this or it would have been very distressing for us both as Steve was unable to lift me.

Lesson learnt - once I get stitches out I'll stick to using the shower until such time I can put weight on my left arm.

Comments

Tracy G (29-11-2015 at 6:20pm)
At least you tried Hun at least you know now .... It's all about finding out what you can and can't do .... I think you're doing fab by the way xxx

Deanna Van der Velde (29-11-2015 at 6:24pm)
You can get aids to help you in and out of the bath. Try Disability North.

Lorna March (29-11-2015 at 6:56pm)
Oh no what a nightmare. I did a sharp intake of breath with my hand over my mouth as I read this post. I was praying you hadn't fallen. Hope you are okay go and have a glass of wine to relax x

Lesley (29-11-2015 at 9:05pm)
I'm sorry ... I know I shouldn't but I did have a chuckle to myself. Look on the bright side, at least Steve was home to help you!
Hate to think what would have happened if he wasn't ☺

December 2015

My first physio appointment.... (01-12-2015 at 12.51pm)
I had my first appointment with the physiotherapist today - not quite two weeks after the surgery. Everything seems to be going well so I've been given another exercise to do and then once the stitches come out I can start weaning myself off the sling. Just for 10-15 mins or so at first, long enough to eat a meal or make a sandwich I guess.

I don't really have any pain as such, mostly stiffness and a bit sore - the right shoulder is giving me more pain at the moment as it's doing all the work and it's a bit worn out anyway.

I plan to go out on the bus tomorrow - what an adventure! I am aiming to go back to work on Monday 14th if everything continues to improve so I need to get used to travelling by bus again.

I will give you an update on Friday once the stitches are out - and if you are lucky you may even get a picture.

Comments

Deanna Van der Velde (01-12-2015 at 1;01pm)
Fantastic Just be careful on the bus it can be jerky

Tracy G (01-12-2015 at 1:23pm)
Wow you're doing fab and I'm so proud of you ....
Obviously your fighting spirit has shone through and you're deffo winning this hands down .... Well done great progress xxx

Lesley (01-12-2015 at 8:53pm)
Wow that's exciting, going out on the bus! I'm thinking that this whole experience so far isn't quite as bad as you'd expected? Enjoy your outing ... hope you're going somewhere nice and not just a medical appointment. It will no doubt do you good to get out the house xx

ME (01-12-2015 at 9:27pm)
I think you may be right Lesley, it's not been too bad so far. I think once I have the confidence to go out on my own with my arm in the sling then things will be easier. Writing this blog and knowing that people care enough to follow it has really helped me. I know that when I have the right shoulder replaced it will be a lot harder as I'm right handed but at least having gone through the surgery and recovery once will help me when the me comes. However, it's all been so much easier having Steve by my side to help me out, he's a total star. ★

Two weeks' post op.... (04-12-2015 at 9.15am)
It's been two weeks since the surgery and I have to say it's not been half as bad as I imagined. I do realise that I still have a long way to go and I won't really know how everything is until I have my follow-up appointment in January, but at least now I feel a bit better about having the right arm done some time in the future. However, I know it will be more difficult as I am right-handed, but at least I know what to expect.

Since my last post I have managed to put on my own socks and a sports bra (front fastening), and put in my earrings without help, and I have been out on the bus and made a sandwich. Such small things I know but they have all been small steps in the right direction.

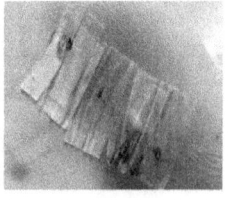
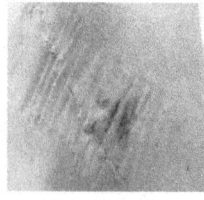

Before Stitches Removed   *After Stitches Removed*

I went to have my stitches out this morning only to find that they used dissolving ones - so it was only the steri-strips which needed to be removed. The lines on the second photo are where the steri-strips were placed and these will soon disappear. I will post an updated photo in a week.

Comments

> *Deanna Van der Velde* (04-12-2015 at 2:16pm)
> *You are doing brilliantly.*
>
> *Tracy G* (04-12-2015 at 4:52pm)
> *So proud of you and I had every faith in you being able to adapt .... You have always been a fighter anyway so well done you're doing fab and well every day is another day towards full recovery xxx*

One small step back.... (05-12-2015 at 12.04pm)

Once more I have taken a little step back. The muscle in my left arm between my elbow and shoulder is extremely painful, which I assume is due to the physio exercises - although I will check on Monday at my next appointment. To make matters worse my right arm is now giving me serious problems again, maybe this is due to it having to 'do all the work'. Getting in and out of bed is a huge effort which means not putting any weight on my left arm, whilst trying not to put too much weight on my right arm - which I can actually hear grinding with the effort. I guess the more my left shoulder improves the worse my right one will seem so the sooner I can do it all again the better.

For those of you who are interested, I have created a Gallery Page showing all the photos from this blog in one place - I will add any further new ones to this page.

Comments

> *Deanna Van der Velde* (05-12-2015 at 4:12pm)
> *Ask the Physio if he/she has any suggestions about getting in and out of bed.*

Claire B (05-12-2015 at 8:03pm)
Sorry I haven't posted for a while, but I have been reading your blog with great admiration and interest. I've heard people who have had a hip replacement say that their 'good' other hip is worse after the op on the bad one, as they're using it more. Apparently you also tend to only feel the pain in the more painful side, but once that starts getting better the other side is then the worst pain and you feel that instead. In any case, you've clearly got a long road ahead of you - but at least you're on it! Get all help you can, and get as much as you can from the physio. It will be worth it all in the end. Take care. x

Physio update.... (08-12-2015 at 2.11pm)

I had my second physio appointment yesterday, everything seems to be going well and my range of movement is pretty good - in fact I can actually reach further up my back with my left arm than I can with my right one. I now have 'level 2' exercises to do and another appointment for 16th. The aching muscles are normal and something which will gradually improve as the strength returns. I have also been given the OK to return to work on Monday, it's only four hours so hopefully it won't be too tiring.

I've been out on the bus again today so it's all practice for going back to work, although negotiating all the Christmas shoppers in town at lunch time when I finish may be a bit daunting. Next update will be on 16th unless any major triumphs or setbacks occur in the meantime.

Comments

Tracy G (08-12-2015 at 2:59pm)
Sounds like you're on track and getting there .... Great news about going back to work and things getting back to normality in some way ... Onwards and Upwards xxx

Claire B (08-12-2015 at 8:05pm)
Great news! Hopefully it was a reassuring appointment as it can be worrying if you don't know why you're hurting or aching a particular way. Hope you have a good week. Don't build yourself up too much about returning to work - if for whatever reason you don't feel like it, don't worry and postpone it. Or perhaps do a shorter day if you can. Thinking of you.

Three weeks' post op.... (11-12-2015 tat 3.29pm)
It's three weeks now since my surgery and so far, I'm very pleased with the way things are going. My scar isn't too bad and the bruises are gradually fading.

Today I wore my jeans for the first time in three weeks so now I'm feeling more like myself again. Jogging bottoms are great when you need the loo and only have one free hand, but now that I'm gradually cutting down sling wearing time I should be able to manage wearing my jeans - as long as I don't wear a belt yet!

I'm now not so scared of having the right one done, now that the left one is almost pain free the problems in the right one seems to be more obvious. Ideally, I'd like to have a holiday in June then have the surgery but all this depends on the surgeon's opinion after my appointment in January.

So I'd like to end by wishing you all a very Merry Christmas and thank you for your support

Comments
Lorna March (11-12-2015 at 4:53pm)
You have done absolutely brilliant, better than anyone could have thought. You also seem much happier than before because of all the pain you have been in its easy to lose the real you. Roll on the next one. Love you lots
Lorna xxx

Tracy G (11-12-2015 at 8:45pm)
Excellent .... I'm glad you're feeling much more positive and your recovery is coming along so well ... All I can say is you are an inspiration and people who search for a blog regarding shoulder replacement will be encouraged by reading yours Shelly.
Well done pet xxx

Claire B (11-12-2015 at 9:16pm)
I'm so pleased that things are going well - you deserve things to go smoothly. You know where I am if you want a moan! x

Lesley (12-12-2015 at 7:11am)
Well done, keep up the good work and enjoy your Christmas xx

Michelle Lester (12-12-2015 at 8:58pm)
Wow Michelle such a big improvement. Bet you really are well pleased with operation. Well done. Looking forward to seeing you on Tuesday x.

Grumpy again.... (13-12-2015 at 9.26pm)
I've got a few aches and pains today, mostly aches in the left shoulder and pains in the right. I'm also having some back pain but I believe this is primarily due to sleeping on my back and struggling to get in and out of bed without putting weight on either arm.

Oddly the bone in the top of my left arm is only now beginning to feel sore - over three weeks after the surgery. I'm not sure if this is normal or not or even if it's something simple like wearing the sling which is causing it.

My neck is once again itching where I had the rash after nerve block was removed and I'm feeling generally anxious and grumpy. I guess I'm now at the stage where I feel I should be doing more and am getting frustrated when

I can't. It's not helping that the weather is turning icy so I'm going to be staying indoors unless I absolutely need to go out. I must try to be careful now as a setback is all I need....

Comments

Lorna March (13-12-2015 at 9:50pm)
You will be fine I have total faith in you. It is only three weeks so don't get disheartened x

Tracy G (13-12-2015 at 10:03pm)
Aww it's still early days like your Lorna says only three weeks so some days good some not so good but stay positive and take each day as it comes as overall you're doing amazing Petal xxx

Lesley (13-12-2015 at 10:27pm)
Two steps forward one step back ... to be expected I would think. Good days and bad .... hang in there ☺

First day back to work.... (17-12-2015 at 4.05pm)
I completely underestimated how hard four hours 'general admin' would be. Although I have been into the office for a few hours the past two Sundays, I did have my lovely Steve with me to help. Today I had to get there by myself, on two buses, wearing a sling and carrying two bags - this was my first challenge. Although I wore my shoulder bag across my body I still had a bag to carry which I had to drop off in town on my way home. I didn't realise how hard that would be. At my desk, I found myself stretching my left arm to pick up the phone and holding the phone really made my shoulder ache. So mid-morning the sling went back on but then I had to stretch across the desk with the other arm, luckily I didn't get too many calls, but everything then took twice as long. I'm not back until Monday so I have all weekend to recover - I don't think if I'd be able to manage a full-time job.

Comments
> *Deanna Van der Velde* (17-12-2015 at 4:11pm)
> *Try and rest over the weekend.*
>
> *Tracy G* (17-12-2015 at 4:46pm)
> *I guess this will be hard but once you adapt and get used to it you will find better ways to minimise the discomfort and awkwardness of everything .... Luckily you're only part time and I hope that you can get used to things .... If anyone can do it, you certainly can .... Rest up Hun and maybe next time you're in you will find it easier xxx*

It hurts.... (18-12-2015 at 6.19pm)

My shoulder was aching a bit yesterday and today it still aches - in fact it hurts! Not sure if I'm better resting it or continuing to do the exercises. It feels like the muscle is stiff and sore so maybe I've just overdone things a bit. I've therefore decided to cut down on how many exercises I do over the weekend and see what the physio says on Wednesday. I'm reluctant to stop doing the exercises altogether as I feel like that would only cause it to stiffen further. So today is another step backwards.

Comments
> *Lesley* (19-12-2015 at 1:51am)
> *Swings and roundabouts .... hope you feel better soon x*

I'm worried.... (20-12-2015 at 7.52am)

After feeling sore and aching on Friday, I woke up feeling much better yesterday. Consequently, I was busy all morning however, when I tried to help change the duvet cover I felt something click and my shoulder has felt odd ever since. I'm not in a great deal of pain however certain movements are now uncomfortable so I had a nap in the afternoon and have had my arm back in the sling ever since.

I had hoped that this morning it would feel ok - unfortunately it still feels 'odd'. I can no longer reach my arm around my back and it now feels considerably weaker than it did 24 hours ago. My worst fear is that something has moved, so until I can ring physiotherapy tomorrow for some proper advice I'm going back to level 1 exercises and keeping arm in sling more.

I'm so annoyed with myself I can't tell you - just when things were going so well too. Might have known it was too good to be true.

Comments

Tracy G (20-12-2015 at 9:28am)
Deffo ring them Monday and see what they say ... In the mean-time try to stick to what you're doing and try not to worry .... It could just be something new you haven't felt before and that's why it feels odd .... I know you're worried you're bound to be but try to settle until you speak to them tomorrow. I'm thinking of you and let us know what the physio says ok Hun... xxx

*Deanna Van der Velde (*20-12-2015 at 11:25am)
Dangerous activity changing duvet covers!

I thought things were going too well....
(22-12-2015 at 3.32pm)

Following Saturday's little 'accident', I managed to get to see both my regular physiotherapist and the shoulder specialist physio on Monday afternoon. After some examination I was reassured that I had really good movement in my arm although one particular area was considerably weaker. I was advised that the joint appeared to be OK but that it would be x-rayed just to be certain. If it was tendon damage, then this would not show on an x-ray but the consultant would be able to order an ultrasound scan if he thought it necessary.

Later in the day I had a call from the shoulder specialist who said that the consultant had seen the x-ray and although the joint was OK, because of the symptoms I had been experiencing he was ordering an urgent scan.

I got a call this morning and went for the scan this afternoon - unfortunately there does appear to be a tear in one of the tendons so I have been called in to see the consultant tomorrow afternoon. Fingers crossed it's something which can be fixed - preferably without surgery.

I'm not a happy bunny - I would say this is a MAJOR SET BACK - I thought things were going just a bit too smoothly. Should have known better. ☹

Comments
Deanna Van der Velde (22-12-2015 at 3:45pm)
Just take it a day at a time xx

Lesley (23-12-2015 at 1:44am)
One word ... Bollocks! Sorry to hear this Michelle ... Bah Humbug ☹

Back to square one.... (23-12-2015 at 4.35pm)
Unfortunately, I need surgery to repair a torn tendon in my shoulder tomorrow morning. I hope to get out before Santa comes but I'm not going to build my hopes up. I'll update when I can. Just as well I wasn't cooking Christmas lunch....

Comments
Tracy G (23-12-2015 at 5:24pm)
Not good news .... I just hope you are out by Christmas and able to enjoy the festive season .... It's been a rollercoaster for you but you're strong and a fighter and I know you will keep on going until you have fully recovered from the whole thing so stay positive and hopefully you will be home for Christmas I'm keeping my

fingers and toes crossed for you and I'm thinking about you Hun xxx

Deanna Van der Velde (23-12-2015 at 6:12pm)
So sorry to hear that. As Tracy said you are a toughie so stay positive and know that there are lots of people thinking of you xx

Lesley (24-12-2015 at 12:58am)
Oh no ... sooooo sorry. Hope all goes well ... thinking of you xx

Christmas Eve surgery.... (24-12-2015 at 4.30am)
It's 4.30am and in three hours' time I will be admitted once again for surgery to my shoulder. This time I won't be staying awake as its classed as emergency surgery so will be performed under general anaesthetic. The surgeon knows of our plans to travel tomorrow morning (4-hour drive) to visit Steve's dad for Christmas Day/Boxing Day and will hopefully get me first on the list. He can't promise to get me out today as it depends on what happens during the surgery - which will depend on how badly the tendon has been torn. The operation needs to be performed within a very small window of time, so if it doesn't go ahead as soon as possible then I may lose full function of my left arm. This is serious and means that I am going back to 'Day One' and this time my sling will be on for SIX WEEKS full-time, instead of the two weeks previously.

I've been lying awake thinking of last time I was in this position - but at least I had time to plan ahead. The freezer was full and I'd sorted out my medication for a month. This time - well it just hasn't happened so once I get home Steve and I will just have to muddle along. Writing this blog will now prove its use to me as I will be reading it back from the beginning to remind myself of what comes next. Although the thought of having to start all over again is unbearable, to go back to not being able to dress myself, put in my contact lenses or cut up my own food after coming so far, is just awful.... and don't even get me started on these bloody awful socks! Another SIX WEEKS of these bloody things .... I was planning to burn them when they were due off on New Year's Eve. I think I will make my new countdown to sock burning day

If it comes to the worst and I don't get home before Santa arrives - then I will see if I can just stay in hospital over the weekend so that Steve can at least go to see his dad. If I'm going to be in hospital, then no point in him being at home on his own so I would prefer he carried on with our plans so that everyone doesn't miss out on their Christmas Lunch. Steve and I can sort out something for ourselves once the real Christmas is over.

So until my next update - keep your fingers crossed for me, and thank you for your support so far on this rollercoaster of a journey.

Comments

Tracy G (24-12-2015 at 10:00am)
I hope everything goes ok today xxx. I know it's a setback and not what you hoped and although I wished this hadn't happened to you I just want them to fix it so you can recover and get to where you need to be so you're fully recovered and able to use your new shoulder as intended. Don't worry about this Christmas Hun you can make up for it next year big style and the most important thing is that they sort this out now and get you home to recuperate ASAP .... Onwards and Upwards Sweetheart it's a setback but hopefully this will be sorted and your recovery will go from strength to strength now with no other problems .... I'm thinking of you and will look forward to hearing it's fixed and you're out of surgery. Take care Hun xxx

Deanna Van der Velde (24-12-2015 at 10:06am)
Hope the blog helps to get rid of your frustrations and that things go according to plan. If you let me know where you live I'm happy to cook something for you both (it's called the Jewish mother syndrome!) Best of luck and thinking of you xx

All done again.... (24-12-2015 at 12.05pm)
All done and back on the ward. Feels like an elephant is sitting on my elbow - it's SO STIFF you wouldn't believe.

It looks like I'm going home later though but I'll wait until I hear from the doctor himself before I get too excited.

Comments
Deanna Van der Velde (24-12-2015 at 12:21pm)
Thank goodness but please take it very slowly...

Tracy G (24-12-2015 at 1:29pm)
Glad you're out of surgery and fingers crossed they let you home xxx.
Take it easy Hun x

Home before Santa.... (24-12-2015 at 9.32pm)
I got discharged a couple of hours ago and seem to have been eating ever since. I'd not eaten for almost 24 hours but wasn't hungry until I started eating. Despite having a sore throat and bruised neck from the tubes used in surgery, I've managed to shovel away quite a few calories - although unfortunately I've not been able to wash it down with a nice glass of wine.

The doctor came to see me afterwards and said the surgery had gone well so now we just have to wait to see how well I will recover. I've to go back to see him in two weeks but in the meantime the sling only comes off to wash and dress and I've to rest as much as possible until then. It's more uncomfortable this time as the sling is tighter and also fastened around my waist as well as over my shoulder but I guess it's a small price to pay if my arm has been saved.

Merry Christmas? (25-12-2015 at 8.23pm)
It's been an odd day, I woke up really stiff and sore - much worse than the first operation, although I guess that the nerve block helped get past the initial stages of pain. We then had over four hours in the car to the West Midlands which was really uncomfortable. I had to sit in the back behind Steve so that I didn't have the seat belt over my shoulder, it made having a conversation difficult - more so because my voice was very croaky because of yesterday's general anaesthetic.

The other thing I didn't realise is that I'd be constantly sliding from side to side so I had to put the arm rest down and wedge myself in with a variety of cushions to minimise any sudden movement of my shoulder. This accompanied by the sling fastened around both my waist and my shoulder, meant it was not the most comfortable journey I've ever had. Fortunately, we are not travelling back for a couple of days so maybe the pain will have subsided a bit by then.

So we will be having our Christmas lunch tomorrow at the same hotel we're staying in tonight, I'll try to get dressed up a bit but to be honest at the moment it's a struggle to get up and dressed!!!

Comments
Deanna Van der Velde (26-12-2015 at 12:06pm)
At least you made it. You are very brave. Hope the Xmas lunch goes well.

A better day .... (26-12-2015 at 9.20pm)
It's been a better day today. I slept ok and we had a lovely Christmas lunch. I'm still in a lot of pain but am reluctant to increase the codeine too much, although I do think I will do that before bed tonight and in the morning, it may make the four-hour journey home more bearable.

It's not been an easy weekend but I'd have been in the same amount of pain at home and at least I got to spend Christmas with Steve instead of being in hospital on my own. The next couple of weeks until I see the consultant are going to be really hard - waiting to know how successful the op went and what the chances are of full recovery. I'm lucky to have Steve with me to drag me out of my black hole in the mornings and to help me through each day.

Thank you all for following my blog, your words of encouragement are a great help.

Meet Nellie.... (27-12-2015 at 8.36am)
I decided that as I'm going to be wearing this sling for the next six weeks, I should give it a name. Meet Nellie - quite apt as I feel as though I'm carrying around an elephant in my arm - or Nellie the noose! I'm also naming the cushion (Humphrey of course) which is constantly by my side. Maybe it's the drugs but if these items are my friends then the least I can do is give them a name.

All ready for the journey home now.... Catch up soon

Comments
Deanna Van der Velde (27-12-2015 at 9:52am)
You've got your sense of humour back Hang onto that xx

Tracy G (27-12-2015 at 12:24pm)
Hope the journey home is not as bad and hopefully once you're home things start to settle. At least you're keeping

*a sense of humour naming your sling and cushion ... Lol
... Rest up once you're home ok Hun xxx*

Square one/day one.... (28-12-2015 at 8.15am)
We arrived home mid-afternoon yesterday after another uncomfortable journey and I was soon reminded that I was back at square one, as I was greeted by all the things that I was banned from doing for the next six weeks. At this point I was wishing I'd not bothered with any Christmas decorations this year, even my half-hearted attempt to 'get into the Christmas spirit' is now another item on the list of things which I need to ask for help with to remove.

I've been awake for a while now, trying to plan how I can get through 'Day One' without losing my mind. I need to take things one day at a time, so if I can get through today then I stand a chance of getting through tomorrow. I understand that I need to (and must) ask for help, but if I can just do ONE THING each day which I can count as an achievement, then I stand a chance of making it.

Comments

Lorna March (28-12-2015 at 10:52am)
You will make it through, you always do. You expected the worse first time around and you managed. I know this time it's longer but it's a drop in the ocean compared to the length of time that you will reap the rewards. IF you behave and do as you're told ha ha. Chin up you CAN do it. Love you xxx

Lesley (28-12-2015 at 2:00pm)
Slowly but surely wins the race x

Tracy G (28-12-2015 at 6:25pm)
Baby steps and no changing duvets. Miss independent is going to have to accept help and like you say do little things nothing major. Lorna's right you can do it and

overcome this setback and hopefully it won't be as bad as you thought. You are so used to doing things and getting on with it but for once you have to learn to ask and accept help Hun .... xxx rest up and use the time to catch up on some TV and reading .... xxx. Once you're back on your feet or arm there will be plenty to do so let someone else take the strain for a while ok xxx you told me to do that and I'm learning to let the lads take some of the pressure off and so must you xxx

Getting paranoid .... (29-12-2015 at 12.19pm)
I'm now beginning to worry about how fragile my arm is, worrying about whether or not my shoulder is being held in the correct position and whether or not the smallest movement may cause another tear in the tendon which was recently repaired. I'm even waking in the morning worrying that I may have had my arm in the wrong position while sleeping - even though I am sleeping with it in the sling every night. If that wasn't bad enough I've managed to bump that arm quite hard this morning and now that it's really sore, I'm worrying more!

I really must get a grip - I'm not seeing the consultant for another week and if I'm not careful I'll drive myself mad. I'm trying to convince myself it was only a bump but the slightest flick of a duvet cover was enough to warrant major surgery last week

Comments
Michelle Lester (29-12-2015 at 2:33pm)
Hiya Michelle, been catching up with last few days' blog. I know it must be so hard especially when you had come on so well but come on girl, head up chin up and that strong brave fighter of a lovely lady will come back slowly I know but you will get there. Off on Monday and Tuesday next week so if you need company just shout.

Love you loads and so proud of you. Keep going you will get there. I know easy for others to say. xxx

Deanna Van der Velde (29-12-2015 at 4:07pm)
Is there no one you could ring to get some reassurance xx

ME (29-12-2015 at 4:51pm)
I'm just being silly, hopefully the consultant will be able to put my mind at rest next week

Tracy G (30-12-2015 at 10:02am)
You're bound to be nervous Petal after what happened with the duvet but I'm sure that if you rest it and don't overdo it and do what the consultant says then you will be ok X. Maybe it's just until it all settles down and no doubt Shelly they have made sure that your tendon is repaired so there will be no repeat of that happening. I guess it's just a case of doing nothing to aggravate it. Try not to worry sweetie I know you're doing everything to minimise the risks now and let's face it you were not to know that would happen but now you do and at least you can avoid doing anything to cause it now. Stay strong ok and try to think positive that it's only going to get better now. Sending big hugs and I hope all the replies on your blog from everyone is making you feel better keep us updated xxx

Good riddance 2015.... (31-12-2015 at 11.57am)
It's the last day of the year and although I could say I will be glad to see the back of it, sadly next year promises most of the same. Two weeks ago everything was going great and it all looked very promising for a good recovery. One week ago I was just coming out of surgery to have a torn tendon repaired, and by this time next week I will know how successful this operation has been (or not).

I'm really feeling sorry for myself today (although I'm trying very hard not to), its New Year's Eve and 14 years since the day Steve and I met. Unfortunately, we will not be in Portugal as usual, nor will we be going out tonight. As I'm unable to put in my contact lenses, I can't even see my own face to put on any make up. I can't have a bath (in case I get stuck) nor can I have a shower as I still need to keep my dressing dry. I'm limited to what clothes I can wear (button up shirts only) and I will be wearing these rotten surgical socks until 4th February. It's also a bit of an ordeal trying to eat with one hand in a sling and I don't want to ask Steve to cut up my food in public. On a positive side, I have been to the hairdressers this morning (as I'm unable to wash my own hair) so thanks to Natalia my hair does look fab

So this New Year's Eve Steve and I will be staying at home, eating party food, drinking wine and watching a film. Unfortunately, due to the amount of pain-killers I'm taking, my wine will be non-alcoholic - but at least I can pretend. Cheers Steve, Happy Anniversary darling and thank you for all your help and support

A big 'Thank You' to all of you too - especially those who have regularly left me words of encouragement, these really do help. I hope that 2016 is a great year for you all and fingers crossed I will be soon on the long road to recovery.

Comments
Deanna Van der Velde (31-12-2015 at 1:18pm)
Happy anniversary to you both xx

Lesley (31-12-2015 at 9:17pm)
Happy Anniversary and Happy New Year Michelle. Try to keep that old British chin up. I feel your frustration across the miles .... hang in there.
Just keep focussing on getting to the end xx

January 2016

Not a Happy New Year.... (03-01-2016 at 1.14pm)
I'm not very happy at the moment, I feel as though Nellie is slowly suffocating me. I have a strap around my waist (my gastric band) as well as one over my shoulder so wearing it in bed means that my ribs ache when I wake up in the mornings. Sitting around on my arse all day is doing nothing for my back problems so last night I had to sit on a dining chair while watching TV - not at all comfortable - especially as I was unable to rest my arm on a cushion as I usually do.

Steve is back to work tomorrow so have to manage without him - although I will get up at the crack of dawn so that he can help me get dressed. I have an appointment tomorrow so I need to go out - I just hope I can manage to get my coat on. The gastric band isn't long enough to go around my coat so I will have to leave it off while I'm out.

We went into the office this morning for a couple of hours just to stay on top of things - Steve was a great help, we got loads done so now at least I don't need to worry about being off sick. I will probably find out on Wednesday just how long I need to be off sick, and how successful the tendon repair has been. To be honest I'm not optimistic of the news being good as it still hurts and it aches like you wouldn't believe. The dressing is still on too, but that may come off on Wednesday then you can have another lovely picture!

Comments

Deanna Van der Velde (03-01-2016 at 1:24pm)
If it helps to get it off your chest, please continue to share xx

ME (03-01-2016 at 1:29pm)
It really does - and it's a reminder to myself for when I have the other arm done. Yes, believe it or not I have not been put off doing it all again - if anything it's made me all the more determined to see it through.

Tracy G (03-01-2016 at 2:13pm)
Hopefully things will start to improve for you Hun ... It can't be easy but your positivity still shines through and glad it's not putting you off surgery for the other shoulder. To be honest you couldn't have anticipated your tendon tearing like it did and unfortunately there is not many blogs on the Internet with this sort of experience so for anyone considering shoulder surgery it's got to have helped them on what and what not to do post-surgery and I know this doesn't help with what you're going through right now but it will help when you have the other shoulder replaced and you will be experienced in the ins and outs so stay positive and fingers crossed it gets better for you real soon. Like your friend says it's helping you to talk about it and get it off your chest. It's not easy but nothing beats the Shelly I know so chin up chick you are an inspiration. xxx

Preparing for the worst.... (05-01-2016 at 9.29am)
Tomorrow I see the consultant but I have the familiar feeling of dread - I'm preparing myself for the worst and I wouldn't be at all surprised if he tells me I need further surgery. My shoulder is really sore today and I feel like at two weeks' post-surgery it should not feel like it does. I fear that maybe I've damaged it again, getting undressed or

sleeping in the wrong position. I'm going to do as little as possible today but to be honest if something is not right with it then rest is going to do little to fix it. I'm toying with the idea of packing my overnight bag now, on the basis that if it's packed then it won't be needed. There is a junior doctors' strike planned for next week so if more surgery is needed I guess it will be sooner rather than later.

Comments
> *Lesley* (05-01-2016 at 10:28am)
> *Oh no ... fingers crossed for you x*

A ray of hope.... (06-01-2016 at 5.23pm)
I had my appointment with the consultant today and despite my fears he is quite happy with my current level of healing. I did express my concern that it is still REALLY SORE, but he said that its only to be expected after two shoulder operations.

My physio starts again next Tuesday and this time I must take it really slowly. I will be back for review in clinic in three weeks but until then I am in the hands of the physio and will take advice from them as to what and what not to do. I completely forgot to ask him if I could try to put in my contact lenses so I will ask that question on Tuesday. However, I have been told that I no longer need to wear the 'gastric band', although the sling will remain in place at least until my next clinic appointment. The dressing is now off and I've been given the go ahead to stop wearing the socks - Yippee! Now I can have a lovely shower. Maybe there is a ray of light at the end of this very long tunnel!

Comments
> *Deanna Van der Velde* (06-01-2016 at 5:43pm)
> *That's much more like it. It can be very frustrating and frightening when you don't know who to ask. Can you not*

give the hospital a ring and ask re your contact lenses surely someone can give you an answer?

Lesley (06-01-2016 at 11:14pm)
Hooray ... glad you can finally have a shower. I was wondering what that aroma was - all the way over here in Oz!

ME (07-01-2016 at 6:22am)
Oi cheeky - I'll be having a word with you later (by email)

More comfortable.... (07-01-2016 at 10.14am)
I'm feeling a lot happier today, I've managed to put my contact lenses in while still wearing the sling - it wasn't easy but now I feel much more like myself. The socks and gastric band have also gone so I'm feeling much more comfortable. My shoulder is still sore but maybe it will start getting better once physio starts. New picture of wound is in the Gallery, and it doesn't look too bad considering it was opened twice in less than six weeks I've not managed to get an x-ray photo yet.

Comments

Lesley (07-01-2016 at 9:38pm)
Glad you're feeling happier. I imagine feeling more relaxed after seeing the doc and knowing all is ok would be helping. Enjoy your snow ... the sun has come out today after five days of rain; not complaining as it's been cold, even had the fire on for our guests who are used to warmer climates – got to a say I was sweating a bit though

Ready Steady Go.... (12-01-2016 at 3.49pm)
Today I had my first physio appointment (again) and although I will be still wearing the sling for at least another three weeks, now I can start to move it. The joint is moving well but the tendon needs to be protected until it has fully

healed so for the moment I have been given just a couple of exercises to do three times a day and then I have a return appointment in two weeks, the day before my next appointment with the consultant. So unless there is anything to report (or moan about) it may be a while until my next post. Thanks again for your support and please pass this to anyone who you think may be interested

Comments

Lesley (12-01-2016 at 9:02pm)
Onwards and upwards .... maybe you could get your next shoulder done in the summer time. At least you could sit outside and enjoy the sunshine! Just thinking ahead ....

Grumpy and Frumpy.... (15-01-2016 at 7.00am)
I'm fed up, I've had a rotten night and consequently I'm feeling very grumpy this morning. To make matters worse I look like a ragamuffin and feel even worse - I'm dying to put on a pair of jeans and a fleece but as I'm unable to put my arm over my head I'm stuck with my checked button up shirts, and as for jeans - well I'm having enough problems pulling up my jogging bottoms with one hand never mind doing up a zip and button as well. Nellie is slowly strangling me and now my 'good'(?) right shoulder is giving me worse pain than ever - serves me right for trying to cut down my pain medication. If it wasn't for the fact I'd probably do myself an injury, I'd lie on the floor and have a tantrum like a two-year old ☹.

Still at least I get out of the house tomorrow when we pick up our shopping then Steve drops me off at the hairdressers - now I just need to find something to do today which doesn't involve using my arms, or my brain, which also seems to have ceased working normally.

>END OF RANT<

Comments

Lesley (16-01-2016 at 3:24am)

Well appearance wise I'm sure you'll feel better after having your hair done (though having said that there's been more occasions than I care to remember where I've felt/looked worse than when I went in!). And anyway, at least you can fit into a pair of jeans! Always a positive ....
☺

Going nowhere.... (21-01-2016 at 8.30pm)

It's been a week since my last post and I'm getting nowhere - literally. Apart from Steve taking me to work for a couple of hours on a Sunday and doing the usual trip for shopping and hairdresser on a Saturday, the only time I've been out is for a couple of hours to the shops with my mam yesterday. Not that I'm particularly bothered, to be honest unless I actually NEED to go out I don't see the point, it's too much effort wearing the sling.

I also feel like I'm making no progress whatsoever with my left arm, two exercises three times a day just doesn't seem enough. I know the consultant said we'd be taking it really slowly but it's so slow I feel like I've stopped, but at least it doesn't hurt any more - my right arm has taken over that role. It's now four weeks since my second operation and I keep thinking of how things were four weeks after the first one - just before I tore the tendon. The improvement was fantastic and I can't wait to get back to that stage again even if it does take longer.

Next week should be different in that I do have a reason to leave the house for most days. Physio on Tuesday followed by appointment with the consultant on Wednesday so hopefully by this time next week things should be moving again. Watch this space.

Comments

Deanna Van der Velde (21-01-2016 at 9:23pm)
Just try and stay positive it's not really been the best of weather to go out xx

Lesley (21-01-2016 at 9:32pm)
You must be up to date with all the daytime soaps by now that's for sure! But I know it can get boring being at home with nothing to do from personal experience. And that's not being incapacitated. Keep that British pecker up Duck!

Good news and bad news.... (27-01-2016 at 5.18pm)

It's time for an update on my current progress, or lack of it as it appears to me. It's so frustrating having to take things so slowly but I understand the importance of it - which is just as well as Nellie is going to be hanging around for at least another four weeks. That was the bad news.

The good news is that both the consultant and physio agree that everything is progressing as it should and its time I did a little bit more. Still unable to wear my jeans though as pulling up is still not allowed with my left arm, so I will just have to put up with jogging bottoms a little while longer. At least I can leave my sling off for short periods while I'm at home but I must keep it on when out of the house - and to take it very carefully when travelling on buses.

I did speak to the consultant today about my original plan (before I had the second surgery) which was to have the right shoulder done in July and he seems to think that this will be possible. My mother thinks I'm a glutton for punishment but she doesn't know how much it hurts.

I'm back to see physio in two weeks and back to see the consultant in four weeks so I will update you with any progress.

I have put my before and after x-rays in the Gallery.

Comments

Lesley (27-01-2016 at 9:05pm)
I was just looking at the photos again and wondering why your forearm is so bruised?

ME (27-01-2016 at 9:28pm)
My arm was held up for the entire operation and then once it returned to the normal position all bruising started to travel down my arm. It was the same thing as when I strained the ligaments in my foot back in September, the doctor told me then that bruising always travels down the body.

Tracy G (27-01-2016 at 10:21pm)
Well that's good to hear things are progressing as they should and although it's frustrating that it's slow better that than overdoing it and things going wrong xxx. Once you're able to get those jeans on you will feel much better and so that's something to look forward to and all this you are going through will be a huge sense of achievement when you finally can use your new shoulder as normal xxx. Chin up sweetie you can do it xxx

February 2016

Insomnia.... (01-02-2016 at 3.27am)
It's almost 3.30am and I'm awake - again, just like I have been for the past three nights. I moved into the spare room over two hours ago but despite all the fidgeting with various pillow configurations I'm still unable to find a comfortable position so I can get some much-needed sleep. Steve has had his sleep disturbed for the last two nights and

has work today hence I made the decision to move beds after my last visit to the bathroom.

It's not my newly replaced shoulder which is keeping me awake, it's the dreadful aching pain in my RIGHT shoulder which is the problem - that and the fact that Nellie is trying to strangle me!

The consultant said that I can start to increase the amount of time I have during the day without wearing the sling, but I'm almost afraid to leave it off as there is a danger of me instinctively using my left arm instead of my right as it's the least painful of the two. I don't know how I can get past this, I want to try to get back to work but how can I possibly use my arms to do four hours at a desk? At the moment I can do the odd hour or so at a time at home but it's so painful.

I desperately need to have the right one fixed however until I have full confidence in my left arm then how can I even consider it? Will I ever be able to reach out and pick something up without worrying that I may have somehow managed to damage something again?

Tomorrow or should I say today, is a new day and a new month although nothing changes. Without having to go to work myself there is nothing to get up for, unfortunately staying in bed is not an option either as I'm unable to find a comfortable position to catch up on some sleep - and so another long day begins....

Comments

> *Deanna Van der Velde* (01-02-2016 at 8:40am)
> *Can you not ring the Physio for more advice?*
> *Remember shy bairns get nowt!*

Moving forward.... (09-02-2016 at 4.46pm)
My appointment with the physiotherapist today was encouraging, I spoke to her about my frustrations and feeling that I'm getting nowhere as I don't seem to have been given enough exercises to do. It will be seven weeks since my second operation on Thursday and I still cannot fully dress myself - although by week 4 after the first operation I was almost back to normal. She explained that we have had to take the first six weeks very slowly but from now I can do a much more varied range of movements and start leaving my sling off for longer periods.

Unfortunately, as my right arm is now giving me so much pain I feel that leaving my sling off puts me at risk of over-reaching, lifting, carrying etc., with my left arm as that one is causing me no pain. So until I am confident that the left one is strong enough to cope I will be wearing my sling whenever I think I need to - the last thing I want is another small movement causing major damage.

So I plan to go back to work on Thursday – it's time I took control of my life back. I realise that I may struggle at first but the sooner I can get back to some sort of normality the better. Sitting around on my arse all day is only making me depressed and giving me sciatica problems. Oddly enough I'm also looking forward to doing the ironing again - yes really - although it will be in short bursts as I need to use my right arm which is the painful one ....

One step at a time, I will report on any progress as and when it happens. Next appointment with the consultant on 24th February.

Comments
Deanna Van der Velde (09-02-2016 at 5:37pm)
Will pop in and say hello

Lesley (09-02-2016 at 8:37pm)
Good on you .... and if you run out of ironing there's plenty over here for you! x

Tracy G (10-02-2016 at 1:33pm)
That's sounds much more positive and I guess it's all down to when your confident to use your arm again. Little by little xxx. I never miss ironing ... I hate it but I suppose if I hadn't been able to do it for a while I'd be the same lol ... Maybe ... Ok well only slightly lol ... Anyway, I'm glad to hear that you can use your arm more and as long as you don't overdo it hopefully this is a sign of your recovery going from strength to strength xxx

A right pain.... (12-02-2016 at 11.40am)
I returned to work yesterday as planned and the morning whizzed past and it was time to go home before I knew it. I was very careful not to stretch for the phone or use my left arm without thinking so there were no problems. In fact, the hardest thing about going back to work was carrying my lunch! Yes, really - with my left arm in a sling, my handbag across my body it left my right hand free to carry my lunch. Who would have realised how heavy a bottle of water and a sandwich could be? My right arm is even more useless today, I feel like I've been lifting weights rather than my lunch. My right shoulder and the muscle down to my elbow is extremely painful and stiff so I'm going to try to rest today. I'm back to see the physio on Tuesday a week earlier than planned due to a change of appointment by the hospital, but before that I will be in the office again on Monday morning - maybe I won't bother with any lunch!

Comments

Tracy G (12-02-2016 at 6:25pm)
*Hopefully it's just until you get used to carrying your lunch ... Or could it fit in your bag?? Glad you're back to work anyway will help to occupy your mind xxx.
Will email you over the weekend x*

Ian (17-02-2016 at 11:45am)
*Every day a little closer from the sounds of it, even if at times it must feel like one step forward and two back. I know that it must be difficult but if you look back to when you first came out of hospital you have made great progress (although not as much or as quickly as you would like). See you for a coffee when you feel up to it.
Regards, Ian*

One better, one worse.... (16-02-2016 at 6.52pm)

There has been a lot of improvement with my left arm since last week's physio session, I've been exercising it regularly and carefully and yesterday I put my jeans on for the first time in eight weeks. I also went to work yesterday although I didn't take any lunch or water - unfortunately it seems to have made no difference as the pain in my right arm is horrendous again today.

My physio is pleased with my progress so it's a bit longer until my next appointment. She is also happy for me to go back to the gym as long as I don't touch the weights! I see the consultant next week so I'll see what he thinks, either way I'll probably wait another couple of weeks. I just wish they could do something to alleviate the pain in my right shoulder until I have the surgery, I'm fed up of all the painkillers

Comments

Deanna Van der Velde (16-02-2016 at 9:17pm)
Mention your right shoulder problems to the consultant maybe some physio on that might help.

ME (17-02-2016 at 6:49am)
If only .... my physio works alongside the consultant and she said not to over work the right one as physio won't help the problem I have.

Time flies.... (22-02-2016 at 3.30am)
Do you know I've now posted over 50 times on this blog, had almost 400 visitors and over 1,500 views? It's also been just over 12 weeks since my left shoulder replacement and just over eight weeks since I had surgery to repair the torn tendon - doesn't time fly when you're having fun.

I'm having another bad night, the pain in my right arm is now constant - like toothache stretching up into my neck and down into my fingers. I'm wondering if maybe there is a nerve trapped in my shoulder. Painkillers seem to make no difference and it hurts whether I use the arm or rest it although it does appear to be worse when resting - or trying to, like now at 3am when I should be asleep. I'll ask the consultant on Wednesday when I see him to see if there is anything which can be done to alleviate the pain until the right shoulder is replaced. If a steroid injection is suggested, then I may just have to risk it although I have been advised in the past to avoid these as they may have an effect on my diabetes - tough choice. Because movements are becoming increasingly difficult I'm struggling to dress myself again. I even left my coat on at work the other day, firstly because the office was cold but then I decided that as I was only there until 1pm it was much easier to leave it on rather than struggling to get it on and off when there was no one around to help.

On the plus side, I'm now only wearing my sling for bed and when out of the house so maybe I'll be able to dump it this week.

I'm free.... (26-02-2016 at 8.27am)
My left arm is doing well and I have been given permission to 'sling the sling' and go back to trying to use my arm as normally as possible. Obviously I need to be careful with some movements and carrying things for a while yet but I'm finally on the right track. It was weird and a bit scary going to work yesterday as the buses were very busy and I purposely carried my lunch in my left hand so that it was not free to grab any poles on the bus. I still need to carry on with physio for some time yet but I need to learn how to use it properly so that it is strong enough to cope when I have the right one done.

I explained to the consultant the problems I am now experiencing with my right arm. Although there is nothing they can do to help with the pain at the moment an ultrasound scan has been ordered to see what is going on in preparation for a second replacement operation later in the year. However, a colleague passed me information about the Paingone pen so I asked his advice about this. I think like myself he is a bit sceptical however at this stage I am willing to try anything so I have sent off for one. It offers a 30-day money back guarantee so I've nothing to lose.

In the meantime, I just need to get on with things best I can. I'm now back to working my two mornings a week and Steve and I have booked a short break next month as I think we both need it. As we missed our New Year holiday it seems like ages since we had a break so fingers crossed the weather stays fine as we are staying in the UK.

March 2016

Getting on my nerves.... (02-03-2016 at 7.34am)

Today is yet another morning when I woke up in agony. The pain in my right arm is constant - over the last couple of days it's begun to affect the back of my armpit as well as my shoulder, down my arm and up into my neck. I definitely think there is more going on here than just osteoarthritis - maybe when I get the ultrasound scan it will show whether or not I do have a trapped nerve. I don't think the pain on the left was ever this bad, and the left arm was the worst of the two before the surgery. Even just after the surgery when my left shoulder was painful and stiff I don't think it was as bad as my right is now - or maybe it's just something you forget.

It wouldn't be so bad if I could at least find one position to put my arm in at night where it was less painful but unfortunately when my arm is still the pain is worse, so often when I wake up in the night it's almost impossible to get back to sleep.

I'm reluctant to try the Paingone pen again at the moment - if it was the planting at the weekend which had made my pain worse, then it would be improving by now not getting worse, I just hope I didn't irritate the nerves by using the pen.

At least now I can get up and have breakfast and painkillers - who knows maybe the postman will bring my ultrasound appointment today.

Comments

Lesley (03-03-2016 at 3:28am)
Aww ... that sounds like a nagging toothache that pain, where you just don't know what to do with yourself ... I'm sorry you're going through this, it's even worse that you live in a country where you have to wait for an

appointment to come in the mail. We moan about our healthcare system over here but if we need an ultrasound, we go and get one ... usually the next day.

More drugs.... (10-03-2016 at 2.30pm)
Since my last update, the pain in my right arm has been increasing on a daily basis, and whilst I cannot say for certain that the Paingone pen is to blame, I can confirm that it definitely didn't help, so it's been returned under the 30-day money back guarantee.

Sleepless nights are now getting more frequent and I'm getting limited in how much I can do with my right hand. Although the left one is improving I must keep reminding myself that I need to be careful not to overuse it. I am concerned that I've been getting pins and needles a lot in my left hand and it's something I will need to mention at my next appointment in April.

The ultrasound for my right shoulder is booked for two weeks' time so hopefully this will confirm whether or not I have a trapped nerve on that side. In the meantime, my GP has prescribed morphine for the pain as I appear to be getting immune to codeine, however before I go down that route I will try increasing my dose of codeine one more time.

All these painkillers mean no alcohol which is not a problem, however I do think it's time pubs started selling alcohol free wine and beer. If it can be bought in the shops why not in the pub? Pubs are selling a larger range of soft drinks these days but as I'm diabetic I find it hard to find any sugar free options so my choice is usually limited to Diet Coke or water.

On a positive note, I did manage to get in and out of the bath at the weekend - one small step ....

Plodding along.... (13-03-2016 at 12.17pm)
It's a lovely day outside, the sun is shining and it makes you want to go outside and DO STUFF. I want to prepare the lunch, put washing on the line, then go outside and spend a couple of hours pottering around in the garden before coming in washing my hair and having a relaxing bath. Unfortunately, what I want to do and what I am able to do are two different things entirely. In reality Steve will put the washing on the line and do the garden while I prepare lunch and maybe bake a pie for the freezer. Later in the day I will attempt to wash my hair but using a hairdryer is out of the question as it's too painful. I can get into the bath but I will spend the entire time in there worrying about how I will get out again. Pain is ruling my life – every morning I tell myself that I won't give in but despite my best efforts I have to limit myself to doing small tasks instead of doing the things I actually want to do. But I'm determined that the pain won't win - everything I do is an achievement.

The link to my blog now appears on the National Joint Registry website under the External Patient Blogs section. It's a useful website for anyone who has or who plans to have, joint replacements so please forward this to anyone you think may find it interesting.

Ultrasound today.... (24-03-2016 at 7.45am)
It seems like a while since my last post, I'm finding it painful to use the keyboard for any length of time as the pain is now affecting not only my shoulder but my whole arm including my right hand. This is a bit inconvenient as I am right-handed however I just keep reminding myself that after the right shoulder is replaced I won't be able to use my right hand very well for some time afterwards so I'm trying to look on this as an opportunity to learn how to do more with my left. The pain is constant during the day

but thankfully taking the morphine at night means that at least I get to sleep. It's not a great sleep as I need to lie on my back, but any sleep is better than none.

I am having my ultrasound this morning so hopefully this will give the consultant a clear picture of exactly what is going on. I may have to wait until my appointment at the end of April before I find out anything, unless the physio can tell me something when I see her in three weeks' time. At least I don't have any pain in my left shoulder, it does get sore but maybe this is something to do with the exercises I need to do or maybe it has something to do with my sleeping position, who knows? All questions to ask the consultant next month I guess.

Quick update.... (31-03-2016 at 2.39pm)
I've been a bit worried about my new shoulder over the last few weeks as it has starting 'clicking' when I move it certain ways. It's also sore when I wake up in the mornings although I'm fairly certain that I am not lying on my side during the night. I'm unsure as to whether or not I should carry on with the exercises and I've not been able to bring my physio appointment forward to get an opinion. So today I thought I would try the impossible and see if I could bring my appointment with the consultant forward instead, although I assumed that I didn't have a snowball's chance in hell. To my utter amazement, I was offered an appointment next week - three weeks earlier than my original date!

So until then I'm going to go easy on the exercises - I only hope that the implant hasn't moved as I don't really fancy another operation on the left arm at the moment. My right arm is giving me so much pain I would rather that the next op is on that arm instead.

On a positive note, at least I am sleeping at night now - thanks to the morphine.

Comments

Tracy G (31-03-2016 at 9:10pm)
Hope all is ok with your shoulder replacement Hun and glad you have managed to bring your appointment forward at least ... I'm also glad you're sleeping a bit better even if it is down to the morphine ... Will email you soon with an update ok sweetie xxx

April 2016

More x-rays.... (07-04-2016 at 7.48pm)
I went to my clinic appointment yesterday but unfortunately my consultant was away so I was seen, over an hour and a half late, by one of his team.

She examined me, got me moving my arm in various directions and said that everything seemed to be looking pretty good but would get x-rays to check and do right one at the same time in preparation for the second replacement.

The x-rays seem to show that nothing appears to have moved but the consultant will take a look on his return in case he wants to have it scanned again. She thinks it may be sore because I'm working the tendon which was repaired and to go back to doing exercises gently and try not to be too concerned about it clicking if it's not painful to move it - which it isn't. However, she also said that as the tendon tissue in that shoulder was very thin, the consultant may be reluctant to operate on it again. So I may just have to put up with it I guess, I'm just pleased I went with the left one first as it's been a really good rehearsal for the right one.

On a positive note, the recent scan of my right shoulder showed all tendons are intact so now that x-rays have been done when I go back on 29th June maybe I can go on the waiting list for the op.

I go back to see the physio in two weeks so hopefully by then the soreness will have subsided.

Cloudy with a Chance of Pain…. (19-04-2016 at 3.57pm)
I've been to see the physiotherapist today and between us we've established that a nerve seems to be becoming trapped during some movements and causing the pins and needles in the fingers of my left hand. In addition, I have had some weakness since the tendon repair but this may be something which will improve over time and exercise. I may need another scan of the shoulder but I'll leave that for the consultant to decide at my next appointment in June. I think the main problem is that I may be getting paranoid - believing that I've 'done something' to it because it's still sore, however the physio said there could be some soreness for up to a year after surgery so not to worry too much about it. Apparently the first 80% of recovery happens in the first 20% of the time but the last 20% of recovery takes much longer. So I just need to be patient, do the exercises and be careful. My left arm needs to be strong enough to cope when I have the right one done later in the year. I'm right-handed so it's going to be more difficult for me to cope anyway.

I've been suffering a lot of pain in general lately - particularly from the right shoulder and I believe that my pain is worse in certain types of weather. So I was interested to learn of the Cloudy with a Chance of Pain project and immediately signed up. The latest issue of the Cloudy with a Chance of Pain newsletter featured a piece on my experience and a link to my Blog, and as a result lots of people got to view it. I would also like to say 'Hi' to my new friend Kelcey in Michigan U.S.A. who discovered my

Blog while looking for info after her replacement shoulder operation two weeks ago. I am thrilled that my experience can now help someone else and that they can learn from my mistakes - which was one of the main reasons I decided to write this Blog in the first place!

Comments

Deanna Van der Velde (19-04-2016 at 4:02pm)
So you are famous all around the world.

Tracy G (19-04-2016 at 5:19pm)
I'm glad that you're progressing even if it is slowly and that they were able to put some of your worries at rest. Hope the trapped nerve somehow untraps itself or at least the physio will help to sort it. I think you're doing great and now your blog is actively helping someone who faces the same procedure ... Well done Shelly x

Kelcey (23-04-2016 at 3:25pm)
Hi Shelly!! Thanks for the shout-out. I wanted to let you know that I am SO happy I found your blog. I am inspired by your story; it sure helps to have someone else who is going through or has been through the same things. You have been a huge help to me during these first weeks of my shoulder replacement. As I told you, you are the VOICE in my HEAD who is always telling me to be careful.... everything that I do, I hear you telling me to be careful! Thank you for being there!

ME (23-04-2016 at 8:11pm)
It's my pleasure, if my experience helps just one person then that makes me feel that writing this blog has done what I hoped it would do when I first decided to write it. Good luck with your recovery.

May 2016

Still paranoid? (05-05-2016 at 8.07pm)
Since my last post I've made no progress, in fact it feels like I'm going backwards. It doesn't matter how much I try to ignore it - my left shoulder hurts. It's one of the first things I notice in the morning when I wake up. I've stopped reaching up with my left arm now as it feels a bit 'fragile'. To make matters worse I've developed a big lump on my elbow, which is probably totally unrelated but uncomfortable nonetheless. I have a physio appointment next week so I'll mention it then, I'll also see if it's possible to get another scan done of my shoulder - even if only to prove I'm just being paranoid. Either way I need to know before I can even contemplate going through with the right replacement - although the movement is getting harder and more painful every day, how would I cope if my left one let me down when I needed it most?

Comments

Deanna Van der Velde (05-05-2016 at 8:31pm)
Wish I could give you some more advice Chin up xx

Anonymous (05-05-2016 at 10:58pm)
Wow this is certainly an ongoing process isn't it? Chin up duck

Another quick update.... (11-05-2016 at 5.54pm)
Just a quick update as there is nothing to report - just more of the same. My physio agrees that I do need some reassurance from the consultant that my left shoulder is ok and as he is the person who can decide whether or not I need a scan, she has managed to get me an appointment to see him next week.

On a positive note, although I've just about given up on the physio exercises, my range of movement has actually improved - just a shame that it doesn't *feel* right.

Moving on.... (19-05-2016 at 5.36pm)
At last, six months after my left shoulder replacement, I feel that I'm moving on, my appointment with the consultant yesterday finally put to rest any worries I've had about my left shoulder not being quite right since the operation to repair the torn tendon on Christmas Eve, four weeks after the first operation.

He is very pleased with my range of movement despite putting my exercises 'on hold' the past few weeks, my x-rays are fine and although it does feel a bit tight and clicks, this may be as good as it's going to get. So I just need to use it normally now and get ready to do it all again with the right shoulder later in the year.

Writing this blog has been really helpful to me, I have made a couple of new friends who have undergone the same surgery and it's been great to share our experiences. Old friends have supported me along the way with words of encouragement when I was really struggling with my recovery and helped to keep my spirits up and Steve has been there every step of the way despite the grumpy cow making more than one appearance!

So thank you all - if anyone is interested in following the next instalment then please sign up for automatic emails for the next update. Hopefully I will have no further problems and the next entry will be the date for my next operation.

July 2016

Update re next op.... (03-07-2016 at 5.50am)

Hi everyone, just a quick update to say that I'm now preparing myself to go through the whole experience again with my right shoulder. Although I'm always going to worry about having to cope with just the already repaired arm; it's now getting to the point where the right arm is so painful I'm unable to use it much anyway. We have been on holiday for a week and the heat appears to have made the stiffness worse. I'm unable to brush my hair or use cutlery and my computer mouse has now been moved to my left side.

I saw the consultant this week and have my pre-assessment appointment booked for 21st July although I'm hoping that I can have the surgery this month if the specialist team are available. Because I have once again opted to be awake during the surgery it needs a particular anaesthetist to be present.

So fingers crossed I get a date for the actual surgery soon then we can start a new countdown.

Comments

Deanna Van der Velde (03-07-2016 at 8:13am)
Thanks for sharing

Anonymous (03-07-2016 at 9:06am)
Ah I was wondering what you'd been up/where you've been ... hope you had a nice holiday x

Lilian Smith (03-07-2016 at 11:01am)
Your bravery still astounds us. Hope you can have your op much sooner. xx Aunt Lil

Feeling low.... (13-07-2016 at 6.27am)
I'm feeling proper sorry for myself today, I slept badly and woke in a lot of pain so I'm sitting up in bed doing emails before I drag myself downstairs to start on the pile of medication. I'm looking forward to the day when I can ditch the painkillers and make the pile a lot smaller but that seems like so far away.

I can't be bothered with much at the moment, my arm is making things really difficult as it's too painful to lift from the shoulder. I'm too busy feeling sorry for myself. I don't do it often so I'm just going to get it out of my system and prepare myself for the next fight.

Comments

Anonymous (13-07-2016 at 7:00am)
Take it an hour at a time xx

Lilian Smith (13-07-2016 at 9:59am)
I'm sorry you are still suffering so much. Not long now though and then you can put this behind you. You truly are amazing to do what you do looking after your Mam the way you do and still going to work. Keep your chin up. Love Aunt Lil

Lorna March (13-07-2016 at 6:48pm)
You have had lots of fights throughout your entire life. You always manage to get through them somehow, I don't know how but you do. I think that makes you more than entitled to feel sorry for yourself, so stop beating yourself up about it when you do feel like crap love you xxx

Your Stories.... (14-07-2016 at 3.25pm)
I've decided to borrow an idea from the 'Cloudy with a Chance of Pain' project and ask if anyone would like to share their experiences of shoulder replacement surgery on my blog. I'm sure that this will be both interesting and

useful, as I myself searched for such a site when I was told I needed surgery and it proved very difficult to find the information I was looking for. So if you can help, please contact me using the contact page and I will publish your story exactly as you give it to me.

I have been sent one to get started so check out the '*Your Stories*' page to read about Peta's <u>two</u> shoulder replacement ops!

The training begins.... (27-07-2016 at 11.52am)
I had my pre-assessment last week so now we wait - and I start to prepare myself for the first few weeks' post-surgery. With help from Peta (who shared her story here recently) we created a list of useful hints and tips which unfortunately I didn't have first time around. So there are now two new pages to this blog, 'Hints and Tips for Surgery' and 'A to Z of Hints and Tips'. If anyone has anymore to add please let me know via the contact page as this can be updated quite easily.

Hopefully I have also learnt how to keep the grumpy cow in check but time will tell.

August 2016

Refresher course.... (07-08-2016 at 7.40am)
I decided to convert my entire blog to book format so that I could read it back easier and refresh myself of what to expect in the weeks to come after my next operation. I must confess that I had forgotten just how difficult things had been so now I am trying to prepare myself more this time. I'm very concerned that my left shoulder is still sore but I am trying to build up the strength by doing some gentle exercises until I see the physio for advice in two weeks' time. I don't have a surgery date yet so maybe I have time to make the left arm a bit stronger before I do.

One of my main concerns is pulling up my jogging bottoms after going to the loo using just my left arm. I am finding this difficult enough at the moment with two hands as my right arm is so stiff, painful and heavy. The action of tugging up with just my left arm causes a bit of a worry as I am not sure how much stress this will be putting on my repaired rotor-cuff tendon. So yesterday I did something really out of character - I bought a SKIRT!!!! Those of you who know me personally will be going - "what, you in a skirt?" I think the last time I wore a skirt was at school many years ago and my legs never see the light of day unless I am on holiday. However, this is a skirt purely to wear at home in the early days after surgery so that I can manage to go to the loo easier on my own. It will probably find its way to the nearest charity shop once it's served its purpose ☺.

Comments

Anonymous (07-08-2016 at 8:21am)
A skirt would be easier to manage, especially if you go knicker-less as well.

700 Today…. (24-08-2016 at 6.32am)

No that's not how old I feel - today I am proud to report that my blog has been viewed by visitor number **700**, this is amazing - thank you to everyone who has taken the time to read this. Secondly, I saw my physio yesterday and expressed my concerns about whether or not the left arm is going to be strong enough to cope when I have surgery on my right, and she gave me some exercises to help with mobility and strengthening. She also reassured me that despite it sometimes being sore, I am doing really well all things considered. My range of movement is very good for a replacement and this had actually slightly improved since my last visit despite just using it normally and not doing any exercises as such.

Because of the increasing problems with my right arm I'm struggling to get myself dressed in the mornings again - hence I feel like I'm on a backward slope. I know that once I get the date for my op I will just have to go ahead regardless of how uncertain I feel about the ability to cope with my left, as the right one is only going to get worse.

Finally, there is another addition to the '*Your Stories*' page, Kelcey from the USA shares her experience of shoulder replacement.

If anyone else wishes to contribute to this page, please contact me.

Comments
> *Deanna Van der Velde (24-08-2016 at 9:22am)*
> *You are a real trail blazer!*

September 2016

Defeated.... (06-09-2016 at 10.51am)
I feel like a failure - after saying for days that I was going to the gym, today I finally went thinking that I would feel better once I'd been. BIG MISTAKE - after only minutes walking on the treadmill I realised that I was going to have to give it up. Not only is my right arm really painful today but I'm also struggling with fibromyalgia. I felt so exhausted I needed to lie on the exercise mat to recover ...... how pathetic. All around me people were lifting weights and running, all I want to do is be able to hang out the washing but I can't lift my right arm so it will be drying indoors again today. I don't give up easily but I realised today that this time I can't win so once I got home I made the call to cancel my membership.

Comments

Peta (07-09-2016 at 10:14am)
Oh dear Michelle. I used to have days like that but please hang on in there.
Things will get better once the op is out of the way. Peta

A new countdown.... (20-09-2016 at 2.14pm)

I've finally been given a surgery date - Friday 21st October - another four weeks to wait, although they will let me know if they can do it any sooner. Now that the date is in sight I'm having a little wobble - because this time I know exactly what is coming and I'm more worried as it's my right arm. Will I be able to cope with just my left arm - especially as it's still sore? Maybe it's sore from the previous surgery or sore due to the fibromyalgia which is causing all sorts of problems at the moment. I bought an electric shoulder pad yesterday after reading about it on the fibromyalgia forum and I found it really soothing, I can use this up until the surgery when I will have to resort to the ice pack.

So I feel that I'm stuck between a rock and a hard place - I know I must have the surgery on my right shoulder no matter what, it's getting more painful by the day and now the weight of my arm by my side causes pain so I find that I'm putting it on my left shoulder quite a bit - maybe it's time to resurrect Nellie ....

Comments

Anonymous (20-09-2016 at 2:36pm)
Glad to hear you have a date.

October 2016

One week to second op?.... (14-10-2016 at 4.04pm)

This time next week I will be in hospital after having my second shoulder replacement - or will I? So much has been going on the past few weeks that I'm wondering if I should try to postpone for a while. My head tells me that's a bad idea as my right arm is getting worse by the day. However, my left arm is also giving me problems, enough to doubt its ability to cope 'on its own' for the next few weeks. Unfortunately, I'm unable to decide if these problems are related to previous surgery or to the fibromyalgia which has been exacerbated by the stress of recent unrelated matters.

My mother has been unwell for some time and I feel like I should postpone the surgery so that I can be there if she needs me - regardless of whether or not I can physically DO much to help. Steve is also dealing with his own stuff and I think it's a bit unfair to expect him to look after me on top of everything else.

So, with one thing and another my head is in a bit of a mess and I don't know what to do for the best, my only plan is to have a chat with the surgeon when I'm admitted and get his opinion.

Comments

Anonymous (14-10-2016 at 4:45pm)
Any chance you could give him a call to discuss things before you actually go into hospital that might help you make up your mind?

ME (14-10-2016 at 5:35pm)
Not really, we had that conversation already a couple of months ago, and he managed to convince me that it's probably as good as it's going to get - in fact he was quite pleased with my range of movement after having two ops

in four weeks. To be fair I'm not sure he could do any more. I guess I'm just getting worried the closer it gets.

Peta (14-10-2016 at 5:33pm)
Go for it! You need the rest after all your ups and downs. Surgeon won't be happy with you if you leave it until day of op and you will deprive others of the slot. It is not going to get any easier if you postpone. The sooner you get on the mend the less work your 'good' shoulder will have to do. Just be careful with the rehab this time. Thinking of you.

Tracy G (14-10-2016 at 6:14pm)
I think you need to have a chat with the surgeon and see what your options are ... after you have spoken to him or his team about your concerns and if you feel like it's not the right time you might only need to postpone it for a couple of weeks .... on the other hand, you have suffered for a long time and the surgeon might recommend you have it as planned regardless of the personal things you have going on but I think talking to him and his team might help you to make your mind up pet xxx. Thinking of you xxx

ME (14-10-2016 at 6:49pm)
We had that conversation already a couple of months ago, and he managed to convince me that it's probably as good as it's going to get - in fact he was quite pleased with my range of movement after having two ops in four weeks. To be fair I'm not sure he could do any more. I guess I'm just getting worried the closer it gets.

Peta (14-10-2016 at 6:56pm)
It is understandable that the closer it gets the more anxious you will be. Plus, other personal complications and health issues I think I too would want to sit in a darkened room and stay there! But you can't! You are no

good to your mother in the state you are now but 4 weeks or less post op, you will be. You have got the freezer full of food so you husband will have the minimum to do hopefully. You need to rest both shoulders which you will after the op - like it or not. You are now wiser on things not to do post op and remember, your first operation was successful: it was getting ambitious post op that caused the problems. And you certainly won't make that mistake again! You will be fine Michelle. We are all routing for you.

ME (14-10-2016 at 8:05pm)
I'm getting some very good advice tonight - thank you all for caring, it means such a lot.

Lesley (14-10-2016 at 7:27pm)
View from across the pond; there is never the perfect time for life's events. There is and always will be something more important standing in the way of our carefully thought out plans. Search your heart, do what you know is best for YOU, and don't look back. At least then, if things go awry, you will only have yourself to blame. ☺

ME (14-10-2016 at 8:03pm)
Hmm sounds like very good advice - you've given me something to think about.
Thank you x

Lilian Smith (15-10-2016 at 4:39am)
Michelle, you must think of yourself for once. This op needs to be done otherwise you wouldn't be on the surgeon's list. Go for it. We'll do what we can if you need us. Aunt Lil.x

One year old.... (17-10-2016 at 5.20am)
Would you believe that this blog is now one year old - how time flies when you're having fun! Who would have thought a year ago that I'd have a paperback on sale from Amazon all about my experience - yes really! Ok so it's never going to make me rich but that was never my intention, however the price is as low as Amazon allows it to be. I'm quite proud of my achievement and I think it's fair to say that I'll be taking it into hospital with me on Friday just in case anyone else is having the same surgery and fancies a read of it to pass the time.

I've got a feeling.... (19-10-2016 at 7.07am)
Two days to go but I've got a feeling that the surgery is not happening this week - watch this space....

Comments

Peta (19-10-2016 at 2:56pm)
Why?

Wandralee (19-10-2016 at 3:56pm)
Shelly, what's happening that you feel that way?

Peta (20-10-2016 at 4:48pm)
Well Michelle. No news so I hope the op is over and gone well. Look forward to an update when you can.

The night before.... (20-10-2016 at 8.55pm)
It's my last night at home before my op - assuming that it does go ahead tomorrow as planned. Before my first replacement I had a feeling that it would be postponed and I was right - and I've the same feeling again this time. Because of this I'm strangely calm - which I suppose is good as if I allowed myself to believe it will happen tomorrow then I'd be a total wreck. Some people tell me that it will be easier second time as I know what to expect but sometimes I think that ignorance is bliss. I'd give

anything NOT to know about all the struggles and frustration that lie ahead in the next few weeks and I'm not sure whether I'm ready to face the Grumpy Cow again.

I feel sorry for Steve who has to live with me and help me as I recover, so I will try not to be an impatient patient and hopefully my recovery will be less traumatic second time round, although as it's my dominant arm I'm expecting things to be much more difficult. My left arm is still sore but whether it is due to the fibromyalgia or past surgery I'm unable to say but I hope that the surgeon may be able to help me with this tomorrow.

I need to be at hospital by 7.30am so I'll be up pretty early, I only hope that I manage to get some sleep. I will update this blog as soon as I know what's happening - if the surgery goes ahead then blog posts will be very short for a while. Goodnight all x

Comments

Anonymous (20-10-2016 at 9:44pm)
Be thinking of you.

Pamela (20-10-2016 at 11:11pm)
Hoping the next 48 hours go smoothly and quickly.

Kelcey (21-10-2016 at 1:38am)
Good luck tomorrow Michelle!! You are a strong woman and you will come through this even stronger, I know this. I've been thinking of you quite a lot lately and will think of you often during your recovery. Please keep us posted as you can ☺

Peta (21-10-2016 at 7:33am)
Well I hope it does go ahead today Michelle then it is done! Having dominant arm out of action it won't be as bad as you feared. That's what I found. I think having had a 'dress rehearsal' on the other shoulder helped! You

have prepared as well as you can. Read your list of do's and don'ts. Take the opportunity to do as little as possible post op which I am sure will help your other ailments too. We are thinking of you.

Now for the hard part... (21-10-2016 at 12.50pm)
Despite my earlier 'premonition' that op would be postponed, it went ahead this morning as planned. I'm back on the ward and feeling ok. Once again I opted to stay awake and therefore was conscious for the entire operation. Didn't sleep at all last night so I'm going to have a nap. Bye for now x

Comments

Lorna March (21-10-2016 at 12:55pm)
Hope you manage to have a good sleep, thinking of you and hopefully the pain is under control. Love you, see you on Sunday.
Take care xxx

Tracy G (21-10-2016 at 1:33pm)
Sending big hugs and deffo time you had a sleep pet xxx

Peta (21-10-2016 at 2:17pm)
Sweet pain free dreams! You are now on the road to recovery! All will be well this time.

Anonymous (21-10-2016 at 2:42pm)
Wow that's amazing try and rest as much as possible. Big hurdle over.

Claire Bradley (21-10-2016 at 6:17pm)
Hi Michelle. I'm thinking of you. Sorry I haven't been in touch before but I've had flu for 2 weeks. I'm glad it went ahead as planned. I think you're really brave x.

Good evening Grumpy Cow.... (21-10-2016 at 4.55pm)
The Grumpy Cow has paid a visit already but she'd better get lost as Steve will be here soon.

I'd forgotten how difficult it was to carry around a bowling ball (nerve block) and what feels like a false arm whilst trying to get comfortable on the bed when the sheets keep sliding and Nellie tries to strangle me. Still it's only for about a month.

Comments

Peta (21-10-2016 at 6:18pm)
Pillows under elbow. lots of them. side bar up to keep them in place.

Lilian Smith (21-10-2016 at 6:30pm)
Glad it's over for you. Hope you're feeling better soon. Love Aunt Lil. xx

Lorna March (21-10-2016 at 9:03pm)
Ha ha you've still got your humour which will help you through. Hope you manage to sleep tonight. Take it easy love you xxx

Kelcey (21-10-2016 at 9.07pm)
Good job, Shelly, you did it! I've tried to leave a couple messages, but I'm doing something wrong. You are a brave soul!!

Anonymous (21-10-2016 at 11:45pm)
Ah it went ahead then! Good it's over with. Lucky we only have two shoulders! ☺

A long day.... (22-10-2016 at 8.30pm)
It's been a busy day with lots of tests going on. The nerve block is starting to decrease so by mid-afternoon I was in a lot of pain. It's also been physically exhausting trying not to use my right hand although I'm pleased to announce that

the feeling has now returned so I'm writing this on my iPod using that hand - well finger really, my arm is still in the sling. The physio is coming back tomorrow to start me on exercises. I hope I manage to sleep tonight as despite my best efforts it's been impossible to nap during the day,

Comments

Anonymous (22-10-2016 at 8:36pm)
Amazing you are managing to write this. Can you not ask for something to help you sleep? xx

Peta (22-10-2016 at 9:49pm)
Hang on in there Michelle. You are one day closer to being better!

Kelcey (22-10-2016 at 11:12pm)
Yay you!! You can do it, grumpy cow or not. You know what is going to happen now (I agree, it I might be better to not know what's coming). But knowing you did it once, you can do it again. Sleeping meds would be my suggestion for tonight! 👍

Second Replacement Surgery.... (23-10-2016 at 11.12am)
I slept better last night (Saturday) so I thought that I'd tell you about my second operation while it is fairly fresh in my mind. Just like last time I opted to have the surgery using a nerve block and no general anaesthetic, so I was awake during the whole procedure.

The nerve block being inserted into the side of my neck just above the shoulder-blade for me (both times) was the most painful part of the whole procedure and seemed to take the longest, although I'm sure it only felt like that to me as various tubes and what felt like miles of tape were applied to my neck and a small amount of my hair, despite it being tied away at the opposite side. Last time the tape gave me a rash when it was removed so this time they used a different type.

The surgery experience this time was a little different. Last time it sounded like carpentry going on in a room next door and I felt little connection to my body during the surgery. This time felt "more involved" as I the screen was clear plastic (although I could only make out the blurry images of what appeared to be a small army, due to the fact I had to remove my specs). I also felt my shoulder being "rebuilt" and the connection of various tools to my body but NO PAIN whatsoever. My arm also felt different immediately after the surgery too. Last time the nerve block left it feeling as though it was pointing towards the ceiling, but this time it felt like my right hand was resting across my body and my "ghost hand" was freezing cold. I also felt as though someone had hung an extremely heavy "fake arm" around my neck and I kept looking at it, touching the hand amazed at how warm and lifelike it was - before remembering that this heavy arm was actually the one attached to my body! As if that wasn't bad enough I was also given a "bowling ball" to carry in a little bag on my left side - this is the nerve block which gets smaller as it feeds pain medication to the shoulder and will be removed on Monday.

In recovery immediately afterwards was different too. Last time I was really cold and they used a warming blanket to raise my temperature before taking me back to the ward. This time I felt fine so I sent a couple of emails to Steve and my sister Lorna from my iPod while I waited to be wheeled back to my bed - they were both amazed that it was all over as they didn't know what time I was going to theatre!

Thankfully by yesterday (Saturday) the "ghost arm" had gone and normal sensation returned to the real one. The physiotherapist has been this morning so now for the tricky part - not to overdo it. I'm finding my book useful as a peek into what to expect next. Although I am also aware that every arm is different at least it gives me a rough guide, whereas last time Steve and I just muddled along the best we could.

If anyone has read my book it is possible to leave review on Amazon, even if you have not experienced it yourself. I'd love to hear your feedback.

Thank you for taking the time to read and for all your words of encouragement. It's taken all morning to type this on the kindle with my left hand so bye for now, more to follow no doubt ☺

Comments

Peta (23-10-2016 at 11:28am)
Well done Michelle. As you say, each op is different. I still don't know how you had the courage to stay awake! Although I had a nerve block with my second shoulder, I was very thankful that I knew absolutely nothing until I woke up in recovery. I must say however that the nerve block was better than a general where you feel woozy for at least 24 hours and going to the loo is an experience whilst still attached to machinery! Any idea how long you will be in? I was in 4 nights first time round but only 3 last time - and I thought that 3 was enough. I was able to get in and out of bed unaided by then and wander around being a nuisance to the nurses!!! Keep up the good work.

Peta (23-10-2016 at 11:30am)
PS are you taking arnica tablets? I found them invaluable to deal with the bruising and my lovely consultant was happy that I took them.

Anonymous (23-10-2016 at 2:33pm)
❀ Brave lady stay positive xx ❀

Going home... (24-10-2016 at 1.27pm)
I'm going home today so I'll do a proper update tomorrow with photos. In the meantime, I'm looking forward to a night in front of the TV with Steve and a pizza, we will do a proper meal tomorrow when we have all day to prepare. So, until then bye-bye. ☺

Comments
Peta (24-10-2016 at 2:33pm)
Yippee!

Anonymous (24-10-2016 at 2:54pm)
Yippee from me too. Enjoy the pizza and the telly x

Claire Bradley (24-10-2016 at 8:47pm)
I am always amazed by your courage and determination! Thinking of you.

Last day in hospital.... (25-10 2016 at 4.18pm)
Yesterday was quite busy. My consultant popped to check on me and said everything looked good and he was happy with the X-ray. I had a visit from two of the hospital physiotherapists who came to check I could manage a flight of stairs and understood what exercises I needed to do prior to my first appointment next Friday. One of them showed such an interest in my book that I gave her the proof copy which I'd taken in with me for reference. She said she thought other patients may find it useful so I also gave her a few of the business card type things I'd made with the blog address and details of book on Amazon printed on them to distribute. I've ordered more copies of the book so that I can give a copy to my physio on Friday. A lady from Pain Management also came to see that I was happy managing my pain and we discussed reducing the meds over the coming weeks. I'm making it my goal to be off the pain medication by Christmas so that this New Year Steve and I can celebrate with a drink together.

Today has been a real struggle, going to the loo or getting washed takes forever and takes so much energy that it leaves me frustrated and getting dressed also takes twice as long. I can only type using my left hand as apart from my physio exercises four times a day and getting dressed my arm must stay in the sling continually for the first two weeks, so blog updates take me ages. My shoulder is really stiff and badly bruised - I will try to upload photos tomorrow.

Comments

Lilian Smith (25-10-2016 at 6:34pm)
It seems that you are doing really well but do try to take things slowly. We're following your progress with mam and hope to see you soon.
Love from Aunt Lil and uncle Peter. xxx

Claire Bradley (25-10-2016 at 8:08pm)
You're getting dressed?! Be kind to yourself and have a pyjama day! ☺ Looking forward to the photos....

ME (25-10-2016 at 8:21pm)
Not getting dressed exactly, just putting something on that I haven't slept in all night. Had four days in nightwear so determined to change into something else if possible :-)

Good morning .... (28-10-2016 at 7.50am)

Good morning everyone - time for a little update I think. For the last couple of days, I've been very busy doing nothing apart from physio exercises, sleeping and watching TV, Steve is home this week so he's been doing the cooking and generally helping with anything I need. I'm sleeping much better and not in any real pain, just very stiff and sore.

This morning I have managed to get my lenses in - HUGE achievement. I also got myself washed and dressed (although I did need help with socks and a belt) ready for my appointment to get my dressing changed. The bruising is coming along nicely so I'll get more photos for the Gallery later.

Comments

Anonymous (28-10-2016 at 8:05am)
Good to hear your news xx

Peta (28-10-2016 at 9:52am)
Well done. Whilst sleeping you are healing! Keep up the good work.

Kelcey (28-10-2016 at 11:29am)
And so starts the healing! So glad to hear you are up and about and still have your wonderful caretaker.

Wandralee (28-10-2016 at 5:33pm)
Hi Shelly! So happy to hear you are doing well.

Lesley (28-10-2016 at 11:18pm)
Great to hear you're doing so well. Hopefully things will continue to improve x

Stiff and aching.... (29-10- 2016 at 10.14am)
BOTH shoulders are really sore today - the left one has been working overtime and the right one is very stiff and aching, so this is all I am doing today, apart from reading and watching TV. I didn't even bother putting my lenses in as it seems less important now that I now I CAN put them in if I want to. So I may just leave them out for the weekend and rest my arms as much as I can. I've put a few more photos in the Gallery and added the option to rate each of the pages.

I'll update this blog later in the week when there is something worth mentioning. Thank you all again for reading and your words of support.☺

Comments

Peta (29-10-2016 at 10:41am)
Very wise to rest. You had more bruising than I did! But it seems to be coming out nicely. It is interesting to watch the colours change over the weeks isn't it? Take care.

Awake again.... (31-10-2016 at 3.54am)

I've been awake over two hours now, the third night in a row I've not slept. At least I'm not in any pain, I think the insomnia is partly to do with the fact I'm doing nothing all day, although I didn't even have a nap yesterday afternoon. Steve is back to work today so I just need to be very careful when I'm on my own that I don't try to use my right arm. The bruising is moving further down my arm each day and the swelling is subsiding, it's aching a lot but not giving me any pain.

I've a friend popping in later, and a pile of magazines and a DVD box set to keep me busy, but it's going to be a long week with only Friday giving me a reason to go out to my first physio appointment.

Comments

Lilian Smith (31-10-2016 at 6:26am)
Your insomnia won't have been helped by the clocks going back. So glad you're not having too much pain. We've been awake for hours now drinking coffee and trying to complete crosswords. We may as well get up and do something useful.
Please let us know if you need anything. Aunt Lil.

Peta (31-10-2016 at 9:47am)
It took me several months to sort out my sleeping pattern after having several months of poor sleep due to painful shoulder, so it is probably quite normal to have a few bad nights, particularly after a clock change. But don't let that stop you taking a little nap during the day - whilst

sleeping you are healing. No sneaky spring cleaning just because you are by yourself this week ☺

Lorna March (31-10-2016 at 6:29pm)
Keep your chin up, you seem like you are doing fine. Just don't rush it, take it very easy with Steve not being there. Love you xxx

Ekidor (05-12-2016 at 3:20pm)
Try and do something useful when awake. It keeps your mind of the fact that you can't get any sleep. you'll naturally find yourself drowsy after you distract your mind from the insomnia.

ME (05-12-2016 at 3:26pm)
I'm sleeping much better now that I've had my op. However, sleeping on my back is not very comfortable and it will be a while before I can lie on my side. If I wake up in the night and can't get back to sleep I just get up and read.

November 2016

In pain again.... (01-11- 2016 at 9.32pm)

For the past couple of days, I've been in pain, especially from early evening into the night. It's not the same pain as before the surgery but it's still awful. At the moment, the pain in my 'new' shoulder is like a knife twisting, and the whole arm aches and I've pain in my right wrist. My left shoulder hurts as though I've bumped it and the muscle in the top of my left arm is painful - probably due to it doing all the work.

Needless to say, I'm not optimistic about getting any sleep again tonight, hopefully the morphine will kick in soon and I'll get a few hours before I'm up in front of the telly again. ☹

A better day.... (02-11-2016 at 4.42pm)

I'm feeling so much better today, it's amazing what a good sleep can do. I think the lack of sleep over the last few days made the fibromyalgia worse; pain and fatigue from this condition on top of shoulder surgery is not a good mix. In fact I'm not having a great deal of pain from the surgery itself, its sore and stiff but hopefully by this time next week it will be much improved. I don't plan on taking any morphine tonight - this is only a 'last resort' when the fibromyalgia starts keeping me awake every night.

I've managed to put earrings in today – three pairs of hoops - as well as my contact lenses and I've had visitors and a sleep, small steps I know but at least they are steps in the right direction. Apparently its freezing outside today, I just hope it's not icy when I go to physio on Friday.

Comments

Anonymous (02-11-2016 at 4:44pm)
Glad you've had a better day

Peta (02-11-2016 at 6:34pm)
So pleased you are feeling better today Michelle. A good night's sleep does healing wonders. So does a bit of "glam" in the appearance department! Ear-rings in was the first thing I did in hospital. I really have quite a silly hang up about not wearing any ear-rings so I approve of making the effort to put yours in. I think you have made very important steps today. Well done!

Wandralee (02-11-2016 at 9:58pm)
I am amazed you can put earrings in your ears! Gives me hope when I have my left shoulder surgery on 11/17. So happy today is going well for you. Take good care.

No physio today.... (04-11-2016 at 3.24pm)

I had a telephone call yesterday informing me that the physio clinic for today was cancelled. Now I have to wait until Tuesday next week so I've decided just to carry on with the exercises I was given, but to increase the number of repetitions until I get new ones next week. Pity I disposed of the exercise sheets from last time or I'd have been able to get started sooner. Still it's probably for the best as I'm keen to avoid any accidents with this one.

I went for my dressing removed this afternoon - no external stitches again however we were very impressed at how it looked once the steri-strips were removed. See what you think - not bad for a two-week old scar. ☺

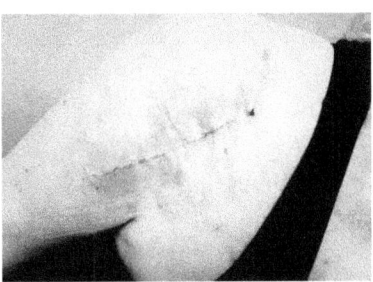

Dressing Removed - 2 weeks

Comments

Tracy G (04-111-2016 at 4:48pm)
It doesn't look too bad Shelly and I think you're right not to overdo things ... hopefully things will just go like clockwork now and as long as you be good and not change any duvet covers it will fly by without a hitch xxx Thinking of you and will email you soon with an update xxx

Claire B (06-11-2016 at 8:34pm)
Hi. The operation site is looking really good, and I'm glad you're feeling a bit better too. You're really brave and have such a determined fighting spirit - keep going!

Taking it slowly.... (09-11-2016 at 2.08pm)

I finally had my first physio appointment yesterday and it went well. Everything seems to be progressing as it should and I've now been given more exercises to add to the three which I was already doing. I discussed my previous surgery with the physiotherapist and the subsequent rotor cuff tear four weeks later and expressed my worries about doing it again. He reassured me that I would be unlikely to do it again having learnt my lesson the first time. So I will be adding the new exercises gradually rather than trying to do everything at once. In addition, I can now start leaving my sling off for longer periods while I'm in the house and use my right hand more. This means that I can now make a sandwich, do the washing up and chop vegetables, although again I will be doing these things gradually rather than trying to do everything at once.

I'm also happy to report that this morning I woke up relatively pain-free and was able to do my first exercises <u>before</u> I took my painkillers. The physio stressed the importance of continuing to take these while on the exercise programme rather than trying to do without them - so again I will be doing exactly as I'm told. My next appointment with physio is in two weeks so unless there is anything to report this may be the last post for a while, although I may add a few more photos to the Gallery.

Today I will be going out on the bus myself as I need to attend an appointment. I have to do it sooner or later so today is as good a time as any. I will get a taxi back though as the buses will be much busier by the time I finish.

Thank you all again for your support and if anyone reads my book please could you leave a review on Amazon? I left a copy at the physio department at the hospital yesterday and they were very interested. In addition, if anyone reading has experience of this type of surgery that they wish to share, please contact me so that I can add it to the Your Stories page. ☺

Comments

Peta (09-11-2016 at 3:16pm)
Continue with the good work. As your Physio said, you won't make the same mistake again about shaking the duvet but don't become so frightened that you dare not do anything in 3 months' time! You really are an inspiration to us all. Well done.

Anonymous (09-11-2016 at 3:51pm)
Glad to hear such a positive report x

Kelcey (10-11-2016 at 12:50am)
Way to go Shelly!! You're on your way to a pain free new shoulder. You are doing great!

Small steps forward .... (12-11-2016 at 9.09am)

I woke up very early and very grumpy this morning as I had an uncomfortable night and Humphrey (cushion) kept falling out of the bed so I had to keep getting out of bed to pick it up, so tonight I will be using a spare pillow under my arm and Humphrey can go on the spare bed!

Anyway, since then I have made progress and managed to eat my cereal with my right hand. This is a BIG achievement as I've not been able to lift a spoon to my mouth for weeks now so it's good to be making a step in the right direction. I wasn't quite brave enough to lift my cup with my right hand though, although I have managed to put on my own socks and put in some hair slides this morning. Maybe soon I will be able to put in a ponytail.

I'm sticking to the exercise programme and I'm happy to report that they are getting easier and less painful every day. ☺

Comments

Lorna (12-11-2016 at 10:24am)
That's brilliant Michelle, sounds like everything is going in the right direction. New year in Portugal could be on the cards if it continues like this. Fingers crossed flower. Keep it going, love you. x

Claire B (13-11-2016 at 9:32pm)
I'm pleased that it's all heading in the right direction. Exercises can be boring but will get you better quicker. Knowing you, I bet you're the physio's best patient! Take care. x

How quickly you forget.... (18-11-2016 at 9.48am)

As I sat eating my breakfast this morning it was hard to remember that four weeks ago I was unable to lift a spoon to my mouth as the pain was so bad - and I realised that I'm heading into the 'danger zone'.

Four weeks after my first replacement I 'forgot' I'd had an operation and with one flick of the duvet cover I was back to square one. I think it's even more dangerous this time as it's my right arm and being right-handed it's only natural to use that arm now that it's no longer giving me any pain, so even though I am now able to leave the sling off for longer periods I shall be wearing it if I feel that there is any opportunity for me to 'accidentally' do something silly. Although my arm is still sore the bruising has almost disappeared and the wound is healing nicely. I will update the Gallery later with photos.

I'm back to physio on Tuesday and I can see an improvement in the movements I've been given so I will probably be moving on to the next level of exercises.

Comments

Peta (18-11-2016 at 4:08pm)
Very wise. Keep up the good and safe work.

Kelcey (18-11-2016 at 11:01pm)
Beware the duvet!! Good for you Shelly, you're doing great!!

Left shoulder one year old.... (20-11-2016 at 12.06pm)

Can you believe that it's one year today since my first operation? In some ways, I feel as though I've been wearing a sling constantly since then and in others the time seems to have flown by. Looking back, it's not been an easy year, the left shoulder having to recover from two operations four weeks apart then having to take over the role as the dominant arm as the right one deteriorated. Hopefully I have now turned a corner, although the left shoulder is still sore one year on, the right one is so much better than it was four weeks ago, before the surgery. My exercises are getting easier and the pain which kept me awake at night has now gone, although the shoulder is still sore and I expect it will be for some weeks yet.

I see the physio this week and the consultant at the end of the month, then I will probably go back to work, although I have been doing some work from home and popping in with Steve on a Sunday last couple of weeks.

It would be great if we could go on holiday for New Year but it depends on what the consultant says on 30th.

How's it going? .... (29-11-2016 at 10.21am)

Tomorrow I have my follow up appointment with the consultant and he will ask me how it's going, so what will I tell him?

Well the pain has gone and I can now use my arm to lift a cup and brush my hair, which is a huge improvement. The wound has healed nicely and the bruising is all gone although my shoulder is still a little stiff but I believe that this will improve with physio. HOWEVER - I still have a lot of discomfort around the back of the shoulder which I thought would vanish after the surgery. I am hoping that this is just because my arm has not been used properly for some time and the muscle has become stiff, I will ask the question tomorrow.

I have been a good girl and although it's getting very boring I have been doing my physio exercises three times a day. Some days it seems like all I do is physio exercises and take my pills but I tell myself that it will all be worth it in the end. HOWEVER - it concerns me that my left shoulder is now giving me problems again. Since starting my physio I have been doing the exercises with both arms and now the left one is clicking a lot more and the shoulder is painful. I know that I'm lucky to be able to use the arm at all after two operations last year but no matter how much the consultant tries to reassure me that it's OK I still feel that something is not quite right.

Overall, I expect that he will be quite happy tomorrow, maybe I'll have x-rays done and be given another appointment for a few months' time, but as long as I can get rid of these awful socks I will be happy. ☺

Comments

Peta (29-11-2016 at 11:32am)
Ah yes - the TEDS. Worse thing about any operation!!! You still haven't let us into your secret about wearing a skirt and not wearing "other things"! You are doing well especially with the physio. Keep up the good work. I am still doing my exercises 6 months' post op - but thankfully not 3 times a day any more.

December 2016

Cautiously optimistic.... (01-12- 2016 at 3.05pm)

My (almost) six-week review yesterday went well with the consultant being quite happy at how quickly I've gone from being unable to lift my hand to being able to hold it vertically above my head. As it is still early days yet he is not concerned about the soreness around the back of my arm and I just have to continue with the physio and ask their advice about when I can get out of the bath etc.

I expressed my concerns about my now clicky left shoulder and was able to demonstrate this quite well as my shoulder obliged with loud clicks on certain movements. He said not to worry about it at the moment as it has been working hard these last six weeks however at my next appointment in three months' time they will get x-rays of both shoulders to see what's happening. In the meantime, it is OK to go away on holiday. ☺

I went back to work today and managed the whole morning without my sling and without any pain or aching. I can leave the sling off most of the time however, it has been advised that I keep it on while travelling on buses and at night for another couple of weeks. Still, at least I got rid of the socks!

My book is going down well at the hospital with both the consultant and physiotherapists agreeing that it is really useful and they are going to pass them around. In addition, I would just like to inform you that this week I reached 1,000 visitors to this blog - thank you all for your support.

Comments

Lorna March (01-12-2016 at 3:26pm)
That is brilliant news Michelle, onwards and upwards from here on in. Now get that holiday booked you both deserve it. Love you Lorna xxx

Tracy G (01-12-2016 at 4:33pm)
I'm over the moon with your progress and it seems your previous experience has made this replacement a much more positive procedure .... I will email you soon Hun but in the meantime, I hope everything just goes from Strength to Strength .... xxx. Great News about your Book and Your Blog I'm sure it's going to help lots of people facing the same procedure ... take care xxx

Peta (01-12-2016 at 4:39pm)
Excellent news. Well done. Enjoy your holiday: well deserved!

Anonymous (01-12-2016 at 5:34pm)
Lovely news Michelle. Now go and enjoy your holiday 😎

Kelcey (02-12-2016 at 12:57pm)
Michelle that's great! Enjoy your holiday and your new shoulder 👍

Bloggz (05-12-2016 at 3:15pm)
Excellent news Michelle. Now it's time to enjoy your well-deserved holiday.

Eight-week update .... (16-12-2016 at 7.32am)

I woke with pain this morning for the first time in weeks. I guess it's a warning that I need to slow down - but it's easier said than done. It's a busy time of year for everyone but why does EVERYONE need to get a bus the same time as me? The streets and shops are crowded and as for trying to shop with one arm in a sling, well let's just say it's no fun. So it's no surprise to me that the stress of attending appointments as well as Christmas appears to have made the fibromyalgia symptoms worse and hence the pain.

Rant over now moving on to the update. My progress is continuing as is the physio, although I can no longer find the time for three rounds of exercises a day at least I'm managing two. This week saw the first ponytail for months as I can now put both hands behind my head. It's just a pity the weather is damp and cold as I'm sure I could hang the washing out now.

I will be having my last physio appointment of the year on Wednesday so hopefully I may even get some different exercises. I'll post an update next week but in the meantime Merry Christmas to everyone - especially those of you who have had replacements this year 🍷

Comments

Deanna Van der Velde (16-12-2016 at 9:35am)
Hope it wasn't the hug you gave me yesterday ☺

ME (16-12-2016 at 9:42am)
Ha ha I'm sure it wasn't x

Ihorse (07-01-2017 8:13am)
Sitting here having first coffee of the morning, reading your whole blog with just over 2 weeks till my shoulder replacement, Thanks. There is so little out there written about shoulder replacements and much of it quite scary. Yours reads as very positive.

ME (07-01-2017 at 12:33pm)
Thank you and good luck with your op. Please feel free to contact me any time before or after your op x

In a better place.... (24-12-2016 at 8.50am)

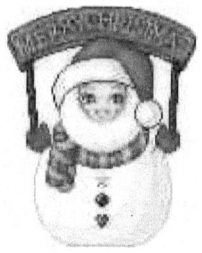

Christmas Eve 2016 is a bit different to Christmas Eve 2015 - last year I was just being admitted for urgent surgery to repair a torn rotor cuff tendon, following a total replacement of my left shoulder only four weeks previously. At the same time, I was also suffering a lot with increasing pain and stiffness in my right shoulder.

This morning I woke without pain in either shoulder and I can now raise both hands above my head with ease. I remind myself that it's only just over two months since my right shoulder replacement and that MUST continue with my exercises for some time yet, however oddly enough the left shoulder is still sore one year after the rotor cuff repair. Both shoulders will be x-rayed again in March so I promise to update again then if not before.

I shall miss writing this blog but I hope that those who have found this useful will keep in touch, especially if you have had replacement surgery yourself.

So for now, I would like to say thank you to everyone who has read this blog and followed my progress through two total shoulder replacements, my surgeon Mr Aldridge and the physio team who have given me two pain-free shoulders in time for Christmas 2016, friends and family, and last but not least to Steve, who has hauled me out of many black holes and chased away the Grumpy Cow on more than one occasion, as well as being there with an endless supply of cuddles when I needed them. ❤

Merry Christmas to you all and best wishes for a better 2017.

🍷 🍷 🍷 🍷 🍷 🍷 🍷

Comments

Lilian Smith (24-12-2016 at 10:24am)
Keep up the good work sweetheart. You are so brave. Tons of love to you and Steve. Merry Christmas and a very healthy and happy new year. Aunt Lil and uncle Peter xx

Kelcey (24-12-2016 at 2:40pm)
Merry Christmas Shelly! Thank you so much for sharing your stories with us. It helped me so much during my shoulder replacement. As I recover from a knee replacement, all your stories are still helping me. My grumpy cow has been visiting me a lot lately, and I can actually smile, for the name grumpy cow anyway!! It makes me laugh ☺. I'm glad you're doing so well and hope everything continues going well in 2017!!

ME (24-12-2016 at 3:49pm)
I've really enjoyed corresponding with you over the last few months. I'll keep in touch then if I ever need a new knee you can give me some tips.
Have a good Christmas and I wish you all the very best for 2017 🍷

Peta (24-12-2016 at 6:25pm)
A positive end to the year and your operations. Well done. Thank you for all your support during my second shoulder replacement!
Enjoy your holiday and continue to have a healthy 2017
Michelle

ME (24-12-2016 at 7:12pm)
Best wishes to you too Peta, I hope we can continue being 'email pals' as I've enjoyed corresponding with you very much and you've helped me a lot with my recovery and the Hints and Tips page of my blog. I hope we can catch up again after the New Year 🍷

Best Wishes for 2017… (31-12-2016 at 1.15pm)

It doesn't seem that long since I was saying *Good Riddance 2015* and here we are again seeing off yet another year. However, in some respects it's been a very long year as I feel as though I've spent the whole year either preparing for or recovering from, shoulder surgery. At least can I start 2017 with two new shoulders, although whether or not that is the end of it remains to be seen as the left one still hurts more than the more recently replaced right one.

So this year I can raise a glass (with whichever hand I choose) to toast the New Year. I wish you all the very best of health and good luck and I will update again after my follow-up appointment in March.

Thank you all once again for your support, please feel free to contact me if you have any experience of your replacement surgery which you would like to include in this blog.

HAPPY NEW YEAR

🍷👯🍷👯 🍷👯🍷👯🍷👯🍷👯 🍷👯🍷👯🍷

Comments

Peta (31-12-2016 at 4:59pm)
Well I think you should put a glass of wine in each hand and practise drinking from them alternately! Well done and I hope that your health continues to improve for 2017.

Today I did my last set of physio exercises and now have good and pain free movement in both shoulders. I will only swim from now on.
So I have put away all my physio equipment. Yippee!!

ME (31-12-2016 at 10:28pm)
Well done you, I do like the idea of two glasses of wine, especially as I've had none all year x

Val (03-01-2017 at 3:09pm)
Glad to hear about your improvement and celebration. I am booked for right shoulder replacement on January 20th. Please God it will take place as I am in so much pain and my arm keeps seizing up. I found your hints and tips very useful and treated myself to some very swish pyjamas! (I'm normally a nightie person). I will keep you posted.
Keep up the good work! Val.

ME (03-01-2017 at 6:44pm)
Hi Val, I will be keeping my fingers crossed for you. Please feel free to email me any time before or after your surgery if you want to ask me anything. Best wishes x

January 2017

Three months after surgery.... (20-01-2017 at 4.25pm)

It's now been three months since my second shoulder replacement and things are looking OK. I've come a long way since this time last year when I was recovering from a torn rotor-cuff tendon on the first shoulder and I had one arm in a sling and the other was giving me a lot of problems - doesn't time fly when you're having fun!

Before I know it, I will have to go through it all again as my replacements may wear out before/if I ever reach the age of 70. However, I am going to be very careful not to do anything silly, I'm still doing my physio exercises when I can and the list of things I am able to do is getting longer each day. Today I reached another milestone by putting my bra on all by myself! OK so it doesn't sound much but believe me when you've needed help for at least two years, to finally be able to do this simple task is a HUGE sense of achievement. I admit I did find an odd way to do it as I can't quite manage to get my hands that far up my back yet, however practice makes perfect so I believe it's only a matter of time. (I put it round my waist and fastened it behind my back and then pulled it up - I did try once fastening at the front and then turning it round but I found that really difficult with two dodgy shoulders).

Some of the other things I can now do include clapping my hands (a round of applause for my surgeon please), raising both arms above my head, putting my hair in a ponytail and brushing my teeth with a manual toothbrush. My next goal is to hang the washing out on the line - however as the weather is rubbish this may be some way off yet.

A couple of ladies have contacted me to say they are soon to have a shoulder replacement themselves so I would like to wish them the very best of luck, one of them has started writing a blog about her own experience. You can follow Sue's blog at https://shoulderreplacementjourney.wordpress.com/

My next (and possibly my last) post will be after my visit to the consultant in March, so goodbye for now and thank you all once again for your support over this last 15 months.

Comments

Lilian Smith (20-01-2017 at 4:40pm)
So glad you're feeling better. Don't forget you really need to look after yourself.
Love to you and Steve.

goggy64 (20-01-2017 at 5:14pm)
Lovely to hear. The future is looking good. I really relate to the clapping comment. Something I haven't been able to do in ages. Feel very rude at times. Post arthroscopies and pre-replacement, my bad arm hasn't got anywhere near bra doing up height. However, with one good arm I can do it up at the front and twist it around. Also, bra wearing really aggravates shoulder - I think it is the pressure from the strap.
Thanks for sharing my blog.

March 2017

The end of the journey.... (10-03-2017 at 5.42pm)

Believe it or not this is the 100th post, so I thought I would give you a few more statistics from my blog to round it all off.

- 5,374 Views
- 1,276 Visitors
- 233 Comments

I have also included a map which shows just how far my blog has travelled since it began in October 2015.

Total Number of Blog Views by Country

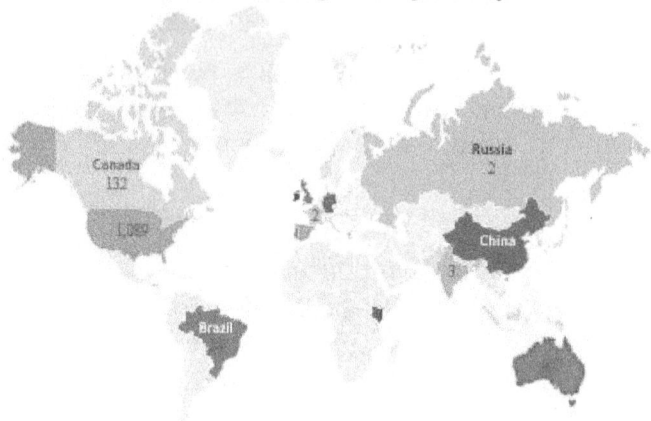

Correct at 10 May 2017

United Kingdom	3,585	Bangladesh	1
United States	1,089	European Union	1
Australia	157	Honduras	1
Canada	132	Hong Kong SAR China	1
Singapore	130	Hungary	1
Spain	94	Indonesia	1
Ireland	61	Italy	1
Germany	51	Japan	1
China	19	Jersey	1
Brazil	10	Netherlands	1
Portugal	9	Norway	1
Kenya	7	Pakistan	1
Cyprus	4	Slovakia	1
Greece	3	South Korea	1
India	3	United Arab Emirates	1
France	2	Vietnam	1
Russia	2		

So I guess this is the end of my 'journey' - yesterday I had my follow-up appointment with the consultant who was most impressed that I could raise both arms vertically above my head. It felt great to be able to hang the washing on the line last weekend after not being able to do so for about two years.

My x-rays were all fine and there appears to be no explanation as to why my left shoulder still hurts over a year since the surgery. It may be because I had a tendon repaired after four weeks, however the consultant is quite happy that everything is moving as it should, so at this stage no further investigation is necessary. I have a further appointment in six months but other than that it's just a case of carrying on with the physio.

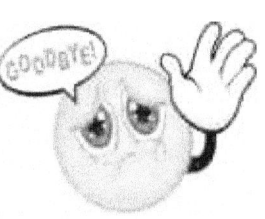

So I'll say goodbye, and thank you, to everyone who has followed me through both shoulder replacements. If you are about to have surgery yourself and have any questions or would just like to contact someone who has been there - please do use the *Contact Me* form and drop me a line.

Comments

Tracy G (10-03-2017 at 4:41pm)
Well done Shelly and anyone reading your blog who faces this type of surgery hopefully will now have a real insight into what to expect pre and post operation xxx

Peta (20-03-2017 at 8:26pm)
That's wonderful news Michelle. Thank you for setting up your blog and helping me and so many other people.

Your Stories

Two Shoulder Replacements – Peta's Story

'You need a new shoulder', said my consultant. 'What?' I had never heard of anyone having new shoulders before. Knees, yes. Hips, yes. But shoulders – no! I had an awful fright. That was in 2012. I chickened out. I had an arthroscopy which gave me relief for two years, but as predicted, I had to return to ask about a shoulder replacement. My lovely consultant introduced me to a lady who had had this operation and we met over coffee so she could tell me about it and show me how successful it had been. Since her operation, she has taken up golf, so I figured that if you could take up such a sport post-op, it must be successful if done by a specialist.

In October 2014, I had a right shoulder replacement and I am pleased to report that this has been very successful. I have 360 degrees of movement in both directions and no pain! Before going for the operation, I saw a physiotherapist and undertook an exercise regime. This was in addition to my daily swim which was by now just reduced to breaststroke (crawl and backstroke no longer possible). There was almost immediate relief from the pain and I was back doing a short gentle swim in just over four weeks and driving (I have an automatic). Exercises were undertaken religiously three times a day, and I made very good use of the ice band recommended by my consultant which had me off painkillers in about a week.

There are several things to consider before the operation of course. Clothing – pull on trousers, button-up tops and button-through nightdresses, and most important 'front loading bras' – very essential when you have an arm in a sling. Being left-handed, I didn't struggle too much with such matters as hair, teeth brushing or eating. I found light bedding best with lots of pillows to rest my arm/shoulder and prevent me from turning onto it during sleep.

I was warned that my left shoulder would need attention eventually. As it happened this was sooner than we both expected due to having had a left knee replacement in October 2015. Why? Well the only way I could get a little bit comfortable in bed was to lie on my left side and of course, I had to use a stick/crutch on the left too.

So in June 2016 I was back for a left shoulder replacement, exactly the same procedure but this time the anaesthetist used a 'block' rather than a general. That was much better but I made sure that at no time was I awake during the operation! The left shoulder was in a sorry state and had started to 'disintegrate' so my consultant had to remove some 'loose marbles'. According to my friends, he is getting to know me too well if he can identify that I have loose marbles! The bruising was much more than before due to the ferreting for the 'marbles' but I am a great believer in Arnica tablets which I took immediately I was awake and continued for the next six days and these certainly helped.

Being left-handed, I was more handicapped than before, but again, I had undertaken some physio, swum until almost the last minute and kept as active as I could. My left arm was 'too heavy to lift' by the time of the operation and I am only now (six weeks' post-op) beginning to lift above shoulder height. But I am confident that I will have the same movement as in my right shoulder once I am swimming again and of course, being diligent with my exercises.

Out came the clothes I needed for the first shoulder replacement: some I needed to start wearing before the operation such as the front fastening bras. I started to practice using my right hand to drink coffee and eat, clean teeth and importantly, getting up from a chair or bed without using my left shoulder at least four weeks before the operation. I have needed more help with other domestic chores and found a tea towel very useful as a bib!!! I live alone so each time, my cousin has stayed to look after me and I have been very grateful for her help and kindness. I started to drive short distances at about five weeks and was helping with the washing up after seven days.

My only concern now that I am pain free is that I will forget that I must not lift etc. for three months and inadvertently use my dominant hand. The right shoulder and knee problems were the result of sports injuries when I was younger so I hope that I will not need any more bits and pieces of me replaced. I have been told that I am already quite valuable to a scrap metal merchant!

August 2016 – Update

It is now eight weeks since my left shoulder replacement. It is wonderful to be out of pain and able to sleep at night. The 'heaviness' in my arm is reducing and I can lift my arm above my head with just a little discomfort. I started swimming about two weeks ago. Breast-stroke only (very slowly) beginning with 10 lengths and adding two lengths of the pool each day. I am now up to half a mile (32 lengths) which takes about 40-45 minutes and I can already feel the benefit of this exercise. I hope to return to crawl and backstroke in about four weeks, again starting off slowly and building up the lengths. I have also continued with the exercises prescribed by the physiotherapist.

Oddly, I have continued to use my right non-dominant hand for many tasks, such as drinking, which is something I would never have done before. I intend to try to continue to use my right hand as much as possible as to become more ambidextrous might be useful in the future as I am 70 years old soon. I occasionally catch myself picking up the shopping with my left arm which I must not do for at least another four weeks. But it is the little achievements which have given me much pleasure. For the first time in three months, I was able to wear stud ear-rings, style my hair and wear a normal bra - though I think I will always have to be a "twizzler" when putting it on!

My Story from Kelcey Michigan U.S.A.

I'm Kelcey, I'm 57 years old. I've been active and athletic my whole life, I've also carried around a bit of extra weight and have a hereditary disposition to joint replacements (my mom has had both knees and one hip done).

At 55, I found myself with a very painful knee and had it replaced. Everything went well.

During this time, I started having pain in my left shoulder (my non-dominant arm; not horrible pain. Usually the pain was tolerable during the day, however, in the evening when I wanted to relax, oh, that's when the pain was bad. X-rays showed bone on bone and I made the decision to have the shoulder replaced.

The first thing I did was some research on the internet. I never watched an actual surgery (yikes!) but watched a couple of YouTube videos to try to prepare myself for what to expect. I found a couple of good tips. I also started practicing using only my right arm for different things. I think that helped me a lot, just doing some practicing.

My surgery was done on a Monday; I was put out for the surgery plus had a block to completely numb my left arm. I am not so sure I would do that part of it again. I have a high tolerance for pain and I think being put out was enough.

The surgery went great; my doctor told me he found bones fragments in the shoulder area that he removed (yikes!). Coming out of the sedation was a bit hard for me this time, but all was well and I went home the next afternoon! Wow- that seemed fast to me but I was very glad to get home.

I purchased a recliner to sleep in and spent most of the first 2 weeks sitting in that chair. Pretty much staring out the front window! I really think I spent most of my first week just getting the anesthetic out of my system. I had books and magazines and my stereo right there...I pretty much did nothing! It was great actually. I spent a lot of time on my iPhone surfing the web; which is where I found the thing that helped me the most.

I honestly don't remember how I found Michelle's blog about her shoulder replacement, just surfing the web I think.

I read about her experiences, how she did it awake (YIKES AGAIN!) and is going to do another one that way. In reading about her experience, what she went through, the pictures......it was so great to find someone going through the same thing. I sent Shelly an email and to my surprise she answered back. I'd get up in the morning and find a new email (we are 5 hours apart in the word) and send her one in return. We conversed this way every day during the time I was off work recovering, comparing stories, commiserating, her giving me the business when I told her I was out on my lawnmower...much too soon in her opinion and she was probably correct!

I can honestly say this was the best thing in my recovery. Using one arm is a pain, healing from having all those muscles and tendons cut is a pain; it's just something you have to get through. Shelly made getting through all that so much easier. I remember when she asked me if the "grumpy cow" had made an appearance yet and I laughed because, yea, that grumpy cow had made an appearance.

Today I had physical therapy and am doing great. I'm back to work, busy as ever. Life is going by so fast. I am not planning to have my other shoulder done for some time, but the time will come. I can't even believe Shelly is having another replaced (and Peta, too, in the two shoulder replacement club!).

Having the down time is great, recovering from surgery is what it is. But having Shelly there to get me through it and keep my spirits up and let me know every day that someone else is going through the same thing, that is the best advice I can give someone who is going to have this done.

The Gallery

Left Shoulder Photos

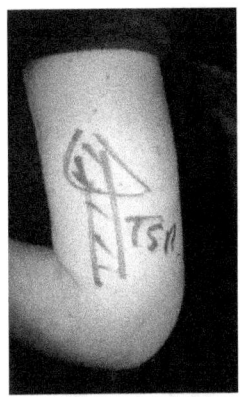

Figure 1: This Way Up!

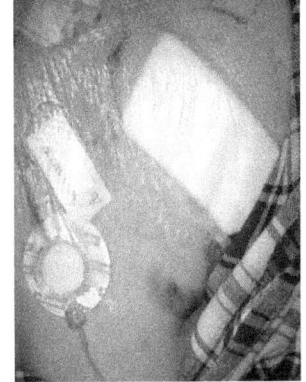

Figure 2: Nerve Block

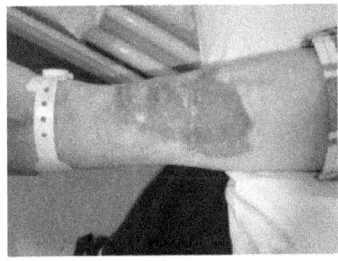

Figure 3: My 'Good' Arm – I Bruise Easily

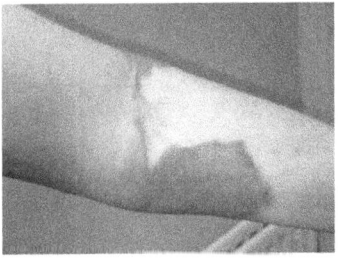

Figure 4: Elbow Bruising

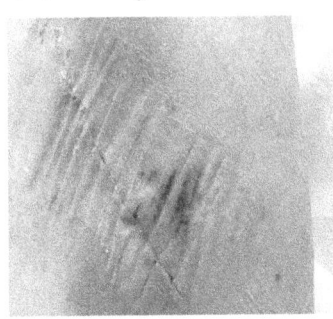

Figure 5: Before Stitches Removed

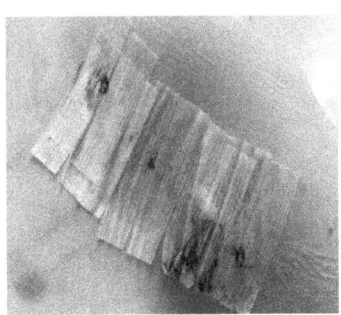

Figure 6: After Stitches Removed

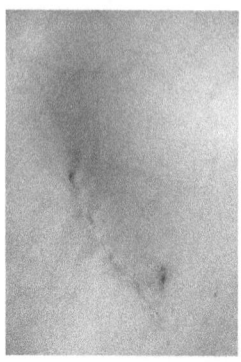

Figure 7: Three Weeks Post Op

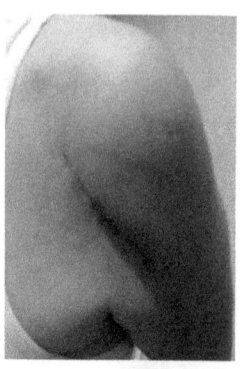

Figure 8: Five Weeks Post Op

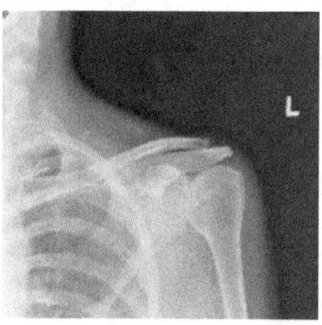

Figure 9: My X-Ray Before Op

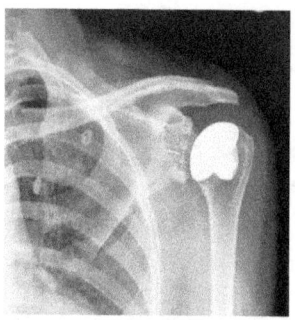

Figure 10: My X-Ray After Replacement

Right Shoulder Photos

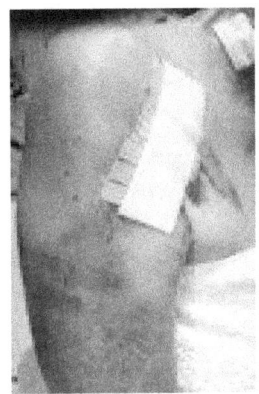

Figure 1: Front of Arm – 5 days

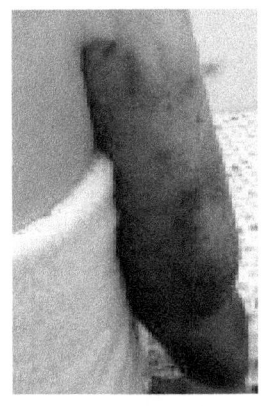

Figure 2: Back of Arm – 8 days

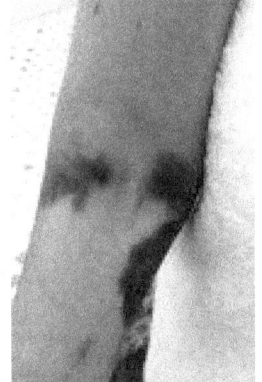

Figure 3: Inner Elbow – 8 days

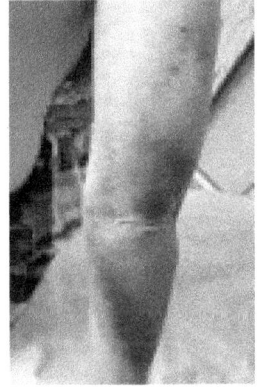

Figure 4: Back of Arm – 2 weeks

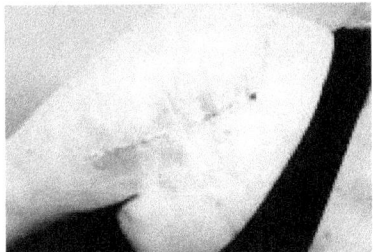

Figure 5: Dressing Removed – 2 weeks

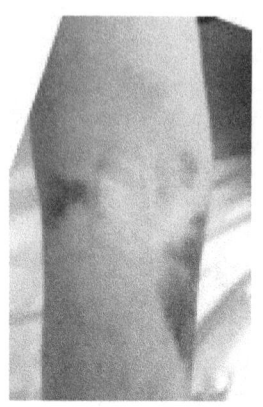

Figure 6: Inner Elbow – 2 weeks

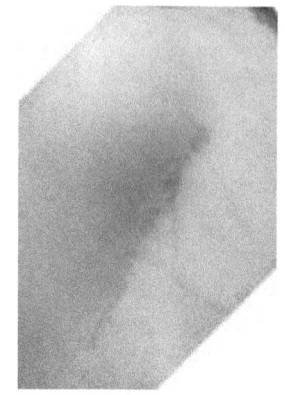

Figure 7: Three month's post op

Latest Photos – May 2017

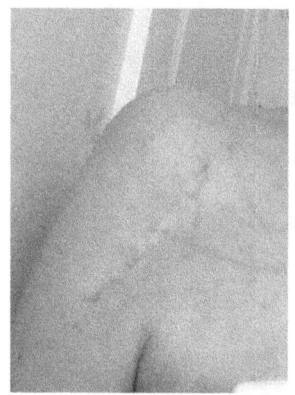

Right – Surgery 21 Nov 2016

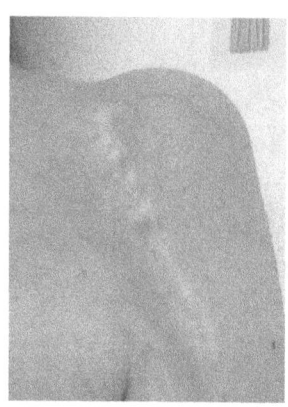

Left – Surgery 20 Oct 2015, Tendon Repair 24 Dec 2015

www.ingramcontent.com/pod-product-compliance
Lightning Source LLC
Chambersburg PA
CBHW070029210526
45170CB00012B/514